KNOWLEDGE ENCYCLOPEDIA

ANIMALS

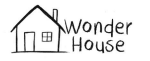

Wonder House

(An imprint of Prakash Books)

contact@wonderhousebooks.com

Disclaimer: The information contained in this encyclopedia has been collated with inputs from subject experts. All information contained herein is true to the best of the Publisher's knowledge. Maps are only indicative in nature.

ISBN : 9789354403958

Table of Contents

Invertebrates

Mammals

Marine Animals

Reptiles And Amphibians

Word Check

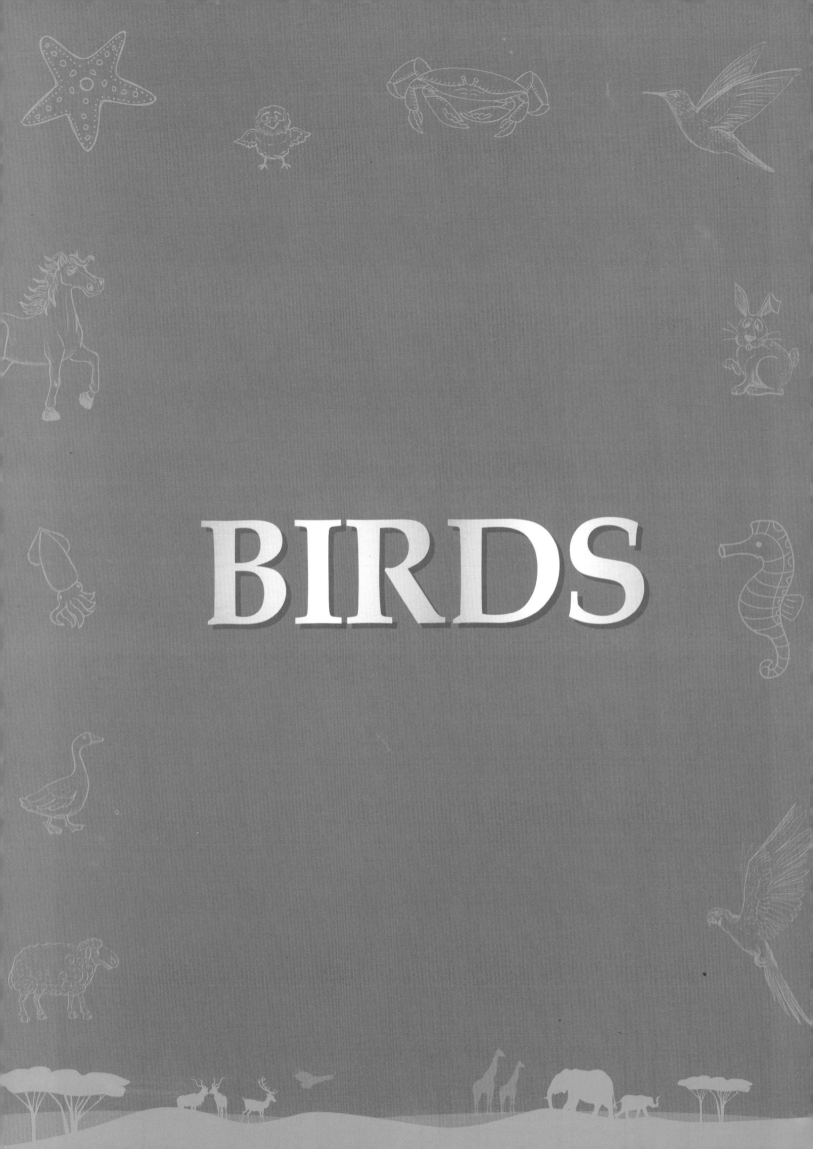

BIRDS

THE INCREDIBLE WORLD OF BIRDS

Did you know that the bee hummingbird is the smallest bird in the world? It is so small that it would easily fit in the palm of your hand! Isn't that amazing?

Earth is full of diverse birds. There are about 18,000 **species** living in habitats ranging from polar ice caps to tropical rainforests, arid deserts, open seas, and mountains.

Scientifically, the entire class of birds is called 'aves'. The name is derived from the Latin word 'avis' which means birds. So, what makes aves special? It is their ability to fly with their wings (which are modified forelimbs). The feathers on the wings help a bird fly. Read on to learn more about the incredible world of birds.

▼ *Birds constitute a beautiful and interesting class of animals that rule the skies*

Birds: Then and Now

You might have seen pictures of dinosaurs that roamed over Earth long before our time. Did you know that scientists have found **fossils** of dinosaurs with bird-like features? This has led them to believe that dinosaurs were the ancestors of birds. It is said the ancestors of birds were theropod dinosaurs. The famous *Tyrannosaurus rex* belongs to the same family.

▶ *Dakotaraptors of the theropod family in a fight during the Late Cretaceous period. Notice the feathers on its arms, tails, and legs*

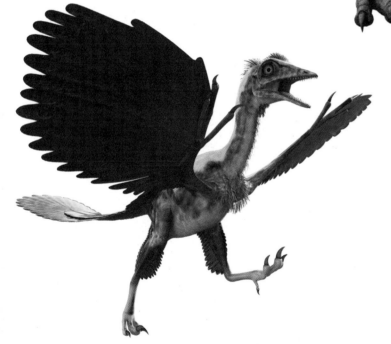

▲ *Modern birds evolved in the Jurassic and Cretaceous eras alongside dinosaurs*

The Missing Link

Have you heard about the Solnhofen Limestone? This is a geographical formation found in Germany. Its speciality is that many fossilised organisms were found here.

In 1861, a startling discovery was made here, which later came to be known as the missing link between dinosaurs and birds. A fossil of a creature named *Archaeopteryx* was found. It was first classified as a bird, but after finding fossils of similar bird-like creatures, it was reclassified as a dinosaur in the 20th century.

The *Archaeopteryx* had small teeth similar to a dinosaur and wings and feathers, similar to a bird. It lived about 147 million years ago in the Late Jurassic period. It was the size of a big hen, but with a light body that could glide through trees.

Incredible Individuals

Sir David Attenborough is a British naturalist and broadcaster. He filmed various animals in their natural environments and educated viewers on how they behave in the wild. He has received several awards for his programmes.

The Modern Birds

As time passed, toothed mouths were replaced with toothless and horn-shaped beaks. The *Confuciusornis* whose fossils were found in China, was the first bird to have this type of beak. It lived more than 100 million years ago and was about 25 centimetres in length.

Another bird-like creature called *Ichthyornis*, which lived 82–87 million years ago, was discovered to have a light skull with a beak. It resembled the modern seagull in how it had strong wings, (possibly) webbed feet, and ate fish. Nearly 66 million years ago, an asteroid hit Earth and wiped out the dinosaur species. However, the early birds, which were smaller in size, survived. This was because of their size and ability to adapt to the environmental changes of those times.

The first modern-day birds called the *Neornithes* emerged nearly 60 to 90 million years ago. In the next few million years, the number and types of birds increased. A journey that is believed to have started over 150 million years ago, culminated with trials and errors to create the beautiful birds we see today.

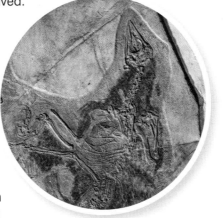

▲ *Fossil of Confuciusornis with a clearly marked beak*

Isn't It Amazing!

About 60 million years ago, South America was an island. This is where the terror birds roamed. One species of terror bird, called *Brontornis*, weighed up to 400 kilograms and ambushed its prey. Another, *Titanis*, could grow up to three-metres tall. With the continental drift, the North and South American landmasses joined at the Isthmus of Panama 2.8 million years ago. Climate change and competition from southward-migrating predatory mammals like wolves and sabre-toothed tigers drove these birds extinct in a few hundred thousand years.

Successful Evolution

When dinosaurs were wiped out of the planet, the mammals were still small and could not compete with the massive 'terror birds' that roamed the land. The birds around this time were so large that some even had a wingspan of 20 ft. The unnamed bird shown here is said to be the biggest bird that ever existed. They might have been the 'elephant birds' who are linked to modern ostriches.

Why were birds so successful? It is because they had the ability to fly. They could take off, successfully defending themselves from enemies. They were also able to reach farther than mammals to find food and shelter. Birds have met the trials of evolution so perfectly that Sir David Attenborough, a popular broadcaster and historian believes them to be the most successful creatures on Earth!

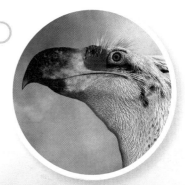

▲ *These scary birds disappeared around 2.5 million years ago*

◄ *Terror birds reached nightmarish proportions, and usually ranged from one-three metres in height and 350–400 kilograms of weight*

A Peek at the Birds

Have you ever observed birds closely? Can you think of all the different parts that give them the incredible ability to fly? Let's find out about all the important parts of a bird's body.

▼ *Macaws are the largest type of parrots*

Warm-blooded

Birds, like mammals, are warm-blooded in nature. Their bodies maintain a steady temperature regardless of the temperature of their surroundings. They do not rely on sunshine to increase heat within them during winter, or on shade to decrease the heat during summer. Usually, their bodies maintain a temperature of 40° C.

◄ *The blue and yellow macaw is found in the rain forest in South America*

Aerodynamics

Birds' bodies are adapted to fly. Their bones are light and hollow. Their legs are held close to their bodies, giving them an **aerodynamic** advantage. Birds have no external ears. This feature streamlines their bodies, allowing them to fly with very little resistance. Also, importantly, birds do not sweat as they lack sweat glands. This keeps their feathers light and dry.

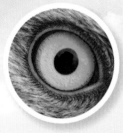

▲ *An owl's eyes are adapted to seeing in the night*

👤✓ In Real Life

The next time you visit a zoo, pay close attention to the owls. Observe their eyes when they blink because they appear to have a third eyelid. This is nothing but a transparent membrane that moves across the eye in most birds. It is called the nictitating membrane. It protects the eyes from injury.

Bird's-eye View

Birds have keen vision, especially birds of prey such as hawks, eagles, vultures, etc. Their eyes help them spot food from great distances. Birds of prey such as the eagle can see as far as two kilometres. Their eyes face forward, which helps them determine the distance between themselves and the prey. Birds that are preyed upon such as sparrows or pigeons—have wider and better fields of vision, as their eyes are on the side.

▶ Beaks are special to birds and they come in various sizes and shapes depending on the food they consume

Beaks and Bills

Birds have no teeth or jaws, but they have beaks, also known as bills. Beaks are primarily used to catch and eat food. They are also used to drink water, feed the young, gather materials to build nests, and for both offence and defence.

Bird Sounds

Can you imitate the sound that a crow or a peacock makes? Birds make different, often melodious, sounds. They make calls, which are short tunes. Or they may sing in long, repeated patterns.

Birds call out when they sense danger from a predator or when they are angry, worried, or guarding their territory. They also sing when they are happy or looking for a mate.

◀ The orange-bellied flowerpecker has very light feet which help it to hold onto branches of trees

Adaptations

Birds have feet which are adapted to where and how they live. A hen has feet suited to scratching the ground to find insects and seeds to eat. Commonly seen birds like pigeons, sparrows, and crows have thin feet with three toes facing frontwards and one backwards.

These types of feet help the bird perch and hold onto tree branches tightly. On the other hand, birds of prey like the eagle or vulture have strong feet with curved talons to kill the prey.

☉ Incredible Individuals

The study of birds is enhanced by artists like John James Audubon (1785–1851) who, in his lifetime, painted a large number of birds existing in North America. He published a book titled *Birds of America* which had seven volumes.

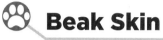

Of Beaks and Birds

Birds use their beaks in many ways. They collect grains to feed their young and gather materials to build a nest, attack and defend, attract their mates, scratch themselves, and also use the beaks for grooming. Beaks can be classified according to size and shape as they help birds follow a specific diet.

Beak Skin

A bird's beak is covered with skin. The skin produces **keratin**, a fibrous, structural protein found even in the feathers of a bird. It is the same protein found in horns, hooves, hair, and fingernails across different species-including humans. The keratin dries up, making the beak hard and tough. It is this protein that gives a shiny appearance to the beak. Few birds like ducks, geese, and swans have a hard, flattened, horny tip at the end of their beak. It is called the nail, and these birds use their nail to dig into mud or swamps for food.

Lower mandible

Upper mandible

◀ *Toucans have long bills that help them attract mates*

Parts of a Beak

The upper part of the beak is called the upper mandible. This grows out of the bird's skull. It cannot move independently. The lower part of the beak is called the lower mandible. It can move independently just like our lower jaw. Beaks come in various shapes and sizes and each one is suited to fulfil the needs of that bird.

Water-sifting Beaks

Most ducks, like the mallard, have a flat, broad beak which they dip into the water. When ducks are thirsty or hungry, they take in mouthfuls of water, which contains food in the form of insects, aquatic plants, algae, and small fish. Their beaks have tiny projections which look like the teeth of a comb. These projections help the duck sort out what they want to eat from the water.

Meat-eating Beaks

Birds of prey like the eagles, vultures, owls, and falcons have hooked beaks. These beaks not only help them to swoop down on the prey, but also to pull off the skin, fur, or feathers of the prey; and to tear apart the meat into small bites which they can swallow.

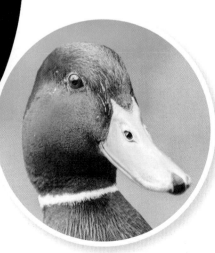

▲ *Ducks have big bills, which is a name for more fleshy beaks*

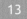

🐾 Nectar-feeding Beaks

Hummingbirds have long, thin, needle-like beaks which they use to suck nectar from flowers. The beak is a protective covering for the tongue inside the mouth. It is this tongue that is used by the hummingbird to pull out nectar from the flowers.

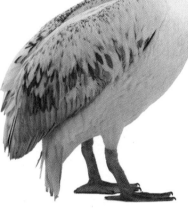

▶ *A pouch-like beak helps capture food better*

▶ *Different hummingbirds have beaks of varied size. The sword-billed hummingbird's beak can go up to 10.2 centimetres, which is longer than its body if you exclude the tail!*

🐾 Fish-eating Beaks

The pelican has a huge beak with a throat pouch. The bird takes in the fish along with water into the pouch. The water is drained out and the fish is swallowed. The upper mandible in the pelican's beak has a small hook-like structure. This is used to spear the fish.

🐾 Fruit-and-nut-eating Beaks

Birds that eat fruits and nuts, such as parrots or macaws, have smaller beaks with hooked tips. These tips are used to rip off the skin of fruits and reach the fleshy and sweet interior. These birds also use their beaks to break tough nuts down to edible pieces.

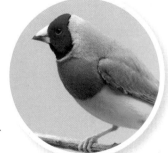

▲ *Parrots are often called 'hookbills', based on the shape of their beak/bill*

🐾 Seed-eating Birds

Seed-eating birds use their short beaks to pick up seeds to eat. Sparrows, like most such birds, have cone-shaped beaks that they use to peck on seeds.

◀ *A beak with a hook gives a good grip to catch prey*

▶ *The Gouldian finch is a seed eater*

👤 In Real Life

Birds use their beaks to feed their young. An eagle captures prey and breaks it into small chunks. The eaglet (as its baby is called) snatches the feed from its parent and swallows it. Most eaglets eat one to eight times a day.

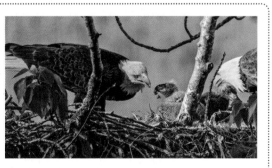

▲ *The baby bird that screeches louder than others usually gets more food*

The Eagle's Prey

A large beak, two heavy talons, and a keen stare—these are the features that distinguish eagles from all other birds. Of the eagles, there are two distinct species that we can see around North America. These are the bald eagle and the golden eagle.

Bald v/s Golden

The bald eagle gets its name from the old English word 'balde' which means 'white'. It refers to the cover of snowy-white feathers on the bald eagle's head. This proud bird is the national symbol of the USA. On the other hand, the golden eagle is the national bird of Mexico. It is the largest bird of prey in North America. It gets its name from the cover of golden-brown feathers on its head.

▶ *The golden eagle can grow to a length of 3 ft, with a wingspan of 6-7 ft*

▲ *The bald eagle approaching a perch to rest upon. This is also how they look when they are ready to snatch a rabbit from the ground*

On the Hunt

Along with buzzards, kites, vultures, harriers, and hawks, eagles are called birds of prey. They follow a carnivorous diet and hunt their food. Eagles can be found in many areas, but they like to live in really high places from where they watch for movement on the land below. All birds of prey have a sharp, hooked curve at the end of their beaks. The upper part of the beak extends over the lower. They also have curved and pointed claws called talons.

Once they spot a prey, such as a fish in the water or a little rabbit burrowing in the ground, they swoop down quickly to catch it with their sharp talons. Eagles feed on reptiles, smaller birds, and **carrion**. Sometimes, they might attack a large deer or even steal meat from other animals.

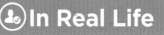 In Real Life

A popular myth says that Ben Franklin wasn't keen on the nomination of the bald eagle as the national symbol of USA because he had learned that eagles like to steal the kills of other animals. However, eagles have long been seen as a symbol of strength, war, and absolute power since the Babylonian era.

▶ *An eagle's grip is up to 10 times stronger than that of humans*

Seagulls

There are more than 40 species of gulls. You can distinguish between them by looking at the spots of colour on their legs and beaks. For example, the herring gull has a red spot on the lower part of its beak. Gulls have strong and gently hooked beaks. They use these to catch and hold fish and water from the sea.

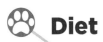 Diet

Gulls are **piscivorous** birds, which means they primarily eat fish. They also enjoy molluscs, worms, insects, and crustaceans. They mainly find food on beaches, but in heavily populated areas they might sift through garbage bins looking for food.

Bigger or older seagulls are so bold that they steal the eggs laid by other birds. The herring gull is known for being a thief. It is seen stealing food from beachgoers and other gulls. It might look for rabbits and even wait patiently for them to peep out of their burrows.

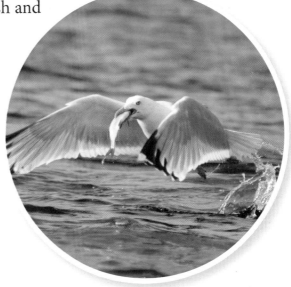

▲ Seagulls can use breadcrumbs to attract fish

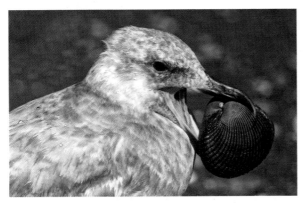

▲ A gull's intelligence is clearly demonstrated in the way they eat molluscs. They drop them from heights to crack the shell and get to the soft insides

☆ Incredible Individuals

Nikolaas Tinbergen (1907–1988) was a British zoologist who studied the behaviour of the black-headed gulls. He wanted to know why they carried eggshells away from their chicks, so he carried out an experiment where he left one set of eggs out in the open and another set of false eggs with eggshells. He noticed that crows went to the decoy eggs rather than the real ones because of the presence of the eggshells.

🐾 Dropped Meals

Gulls enjoy molluscs and crustaceans, but they have hard shells. So, how do the birds eat them? Cleverly, the gulls carry these molluscs in their beaks as they fly and drop them from a height onto hard rocks so that their shells crack.

🐾 Intelligent Behaviour

Gulls are highly intelligent birds. The black-headed gulls practice an interesting method called 'eggshell removal'. After their eggs hatch, these gulls rush to move the eggshells far away from the newly hatched chicks. This practice protects the chicks from getting injured by the sharp edges of the broken eggshells.

This removal also prevents predators like the herring gulls and crows from preying on the chicks. The insides of the eggs, which have certain odours, attract these predators. When these eggshells are moved away, the predators fly towards the eggshells, leaving the chicks safe.

▲ Some studies show that if you stare them down, seagulls will hesitate a little longer before grabbing your French fry

The Filtering Flamingo

A group of flamingos is called a flock or flamboyance. If you live in South America, Africa, or certain parts of Europe and Asia, you have probably seen these flamboyant birds. They have long, slender, and curved necks and wide, flat black-tipped beaks. The pink feathers that cover their bodies are their most unique feature.

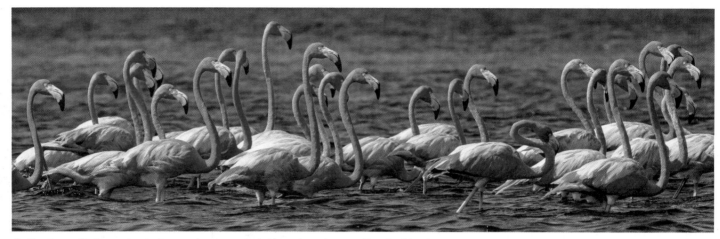

▲ Flamingos flock together in thousands near water bodies where they can filter-feed for shrimp, algae, and insects

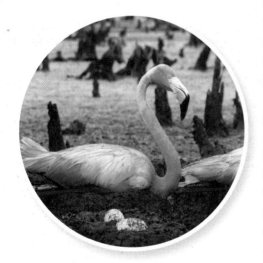

▲ Male and female flamingos build a nest together and both sit on the egg while it incubates for about a month

🐾 Social Habits

It is rare to see a flamingo on its own, as it is an extremely social bird. They are seen in groups of hundreds or even millions near lakes. They keep themselves warm by standing on one leg, keeping the raised leg dry. These birds build their nests out of the mud available on the shores. They stack up the mud in the shape of a cone until it stands several inches above the ground. It is here that they lay their eggs.

🐾 Diet

Flamingos feed by bending their long necks down and pushing their beaks underwater. They disturb the ground beneath the water by moving their feet, shuffling the organic matter about. This ruffles up delicious servings of plankton, algae, small fish, larvae, and mini-invertebrates such as crustaceans and molluscs.

Unfortunately, they also catch some muddy water in their beaks along with the food. So, they simply move their heads side-to-side to filter out the water. Their short beaks have small structures within, which help this process along. Then, they simply expel the water from their beaks. Ducks and swans also possess this filtering ability.

👤✓ In Real Life

The flashy pink colour of the flamingos' feathers comes from their diet. Baby flamingos are born with a white or grey plumage that only turns pink after two years of eating food that contains carotenoid pigments. Flamingos in zoos consume food colouring so that this pink colour does not fade.

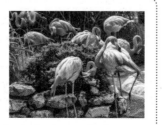

▲ The feathers under flamingos' wings are black

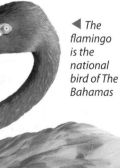

◀ The flamingo is the national bird of The Bahamas

The Wading Stork

In many countries, children are told that they were delivered to their parents by the stork. The image is always of a stork with its almost-straight beak carrying a baby wrapped within a blanket. In reality, storks use their long beaks to fish for food and communicate by making a bill-clattering noise that sounds like distant machine-gun fire.

▼ *The myth can be traced back to Greek roots, where Hera changed one of Zeus's lovers into a stork as revenge*

Fishing Time

Storks prefer to feed during the day and like to catch fish and other small animals. Some only eat carrion. When storks feel hungry, they fly above water with their beaks open. They put their beaks in the water and appear to walk above the surface. As soon as a fish gets close to the beak, the storks close it. They take as little as 25 milliseconds to do this, so the poor trapped fish cannot escape. As a result of this remarkable feeding habit, storks are called wading birds. They are seen moving and even standing still in the water. The spoonbill is another example of a wading bird.

▲ *A stork approaching the water to begin feeding*

Storks usually wade above freshwater lakes and ponds where there are plenty of fish. They are seen in the warmer areas of Asia, Africa, and Europe. They like to feed in flocks as they love being around other storks. During the breeding season they break into pairs—each pair happily eating around 180 kilograms of fish in one season.

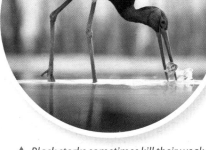

▲ *Black storks sometimes kill their weak babies when there is shortage of food*

Isn't It Amazing!

Storks do not have a vocal organ or 'syrinx', so they do not have a call like most other birds. Instead, if they want to make a sound, they clatter their beaks in different ways to share a feeling of excitement.

Incredible Individuals

India and Cambodia have seen a decline in their number of storks due to deforestation. Unhappy with this development, a group of 70 women from Assam, India formed the Hargilla Army. (Hargilla is the name given to storks in Sanskrit.)

Storks build nesting trees which were lost after deforestation. They also suffered from the poor impression they made on the locals because of their smell and large size. So, the Hargilla Army educated people about the importance of storks and protecting the trees, making sure that no more nesting trees were cut down since 2010.

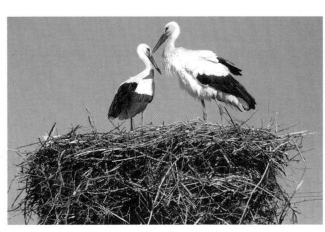

▲ *Storks are known to stay and continue breeding in one nest for many years*

Red Robins

There are two main species of robins; they are the American robin and the European robin. The American robin is bigger, with a length of 25 centimetres while the European robin is around 10 centimetres. They can be distinguished by the colour of the feathers on their breast—rusty red if American, and scarlet orange if European.

◀ *American robin is the state bird for Connecticut, Michigan, and Wisconsin*

▶ *European robin can cope with cold and snow, but far northern Europe can still be too much*

Diet

American robins prefer to feed on a diet of small insects, earthworms, and delicious berries. European robins mainly eat insects like grasshoppers and caterpillars. Both species like to look for food during the day. European robins live in suburban areas and follow gardeners. As the gardener goes about digging the ground, the robin quickly grabs any insect that might be disturbed from the soil. Similarly, American robins spend most of their day hopping around on grass, looking for earthworms.

Feeding Habits

Robins have thin, straight beaks that are quite small. Other insect-eating birds like swallows might fly close to the ground with their beaks apart, ready to catch an insect whether it is stationary or moving. On the other hand, robins prefer to catch insects while standing in one place. They practice a run-and-stop technique to catch their food. Robins also rest on the branches of trees and pluck berries individually with their beaks.

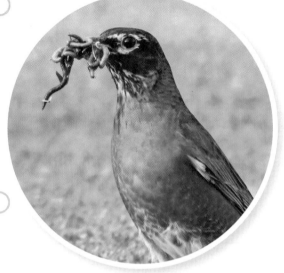

▲ *If there is a choice of foods, most robins prefer meal worms above other things*

▼ *Each robin has a unique breast pattern and can be recognised individually*

The Songbird

Robins, like sparrows, live in populated areas and do not mind the presence of human beings. They have sweet, melodious voices, and they sing to other birds to communicate and mate. The European robin tends to emit high-pitched notes throughout the year. The American robins sing before and after sunrise. They only repeat two or three 'syllables' when they sing but it is cheery and pleasant to hear.

▶ *Both male and female robins sing the same winter song*

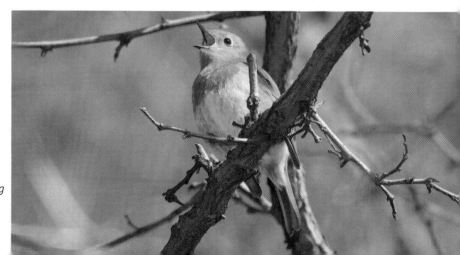

The Sparrow's Seeds

Sparrows are such a common sight, they seem like the most common bird in the world. One of their species, the house sparrows, are the most widely seen in the world. These birds, along with goldfinches, are seed- and grain-eating birds.

House Sparrows

House sparrows, like all other sparrows, have short and cone-shaped beaks. They use these to break the seeds and eat them. Their legs are short. Though they are small and just around 15 centimetres in length, these birds have stout bodies. They are often on the lookout for any crumbs of food they can find. They might even steal from other birds like the American robin.

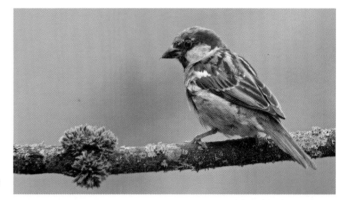

▶ *House sparrows just weigh around 30 grams*

Lark Sparrows

Lark sparrows like to roam along sandy or barren lands to find seeds or grains. They are about the same size as the house sparrow. As soon as they feel too warm or sense a threat, they find a tall perch to sit on. These birds avoid confrontation. They might fly away in a hurry if they are approached by human beings.

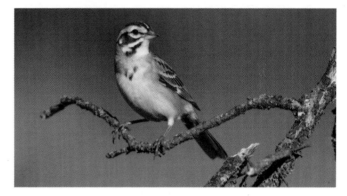

▶ *The harlequin facial pattern and white tail spots make the lark sparrow standout among sparrows*

Golden-Crowned Sparrows

The golden-crowned sparrows get their name from the small patch of yellow plumage visible at the top of their crown or head. During the winter season, these sparrows join the flock of the other sparrow species for protection. These birds eat seeds from fruits and flowers in open garden areas. They also happily nip at vegetables like peas, beets, and cabbages.

Golden-crowned sparrows can be seen in the fall and spring seasons in shrubs and weeds. The birds use their beaks to scratch leaves or peck on them to find seeds. They are often spotted hopping on the ground.

▶ *The call of a golden-crowned sparrow sounds like a whistle*

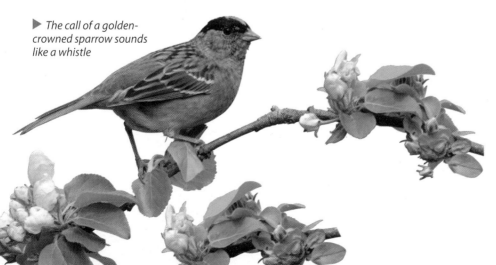

Fox Sparrows

Fox sparrows are seen in places where there is thick shrubbery or plant cover. They like to eat small seeds that they might find on the ground. They also eat small berries. They might be seen scratching up bird feeders that people have left out. These sparrows are named for their reddish plumage. However, while some birds have the fox-like red covering, other birds might display a dark brown or even grey cover of feathers.

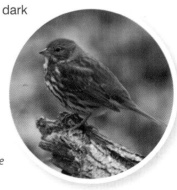

▶ *Fox sparrows spend a lot of time on the ground*

The Macaw's Fruit

Macaws belong to the parrot family. There are 18 different species found in North and South America. A unique thing about macaws is that despite being a colourful species, both the male and female look like each other.

◀ *A macaw grips the fruit with its toes*

Beaks and Skills

Macaws have curved, sickle-shaped beaks where the upper part of the beak extends over the lower. These beaks are big enough to hold nuts in, and strong enough to crack them apart with little effort. The macaws also have strong, muscly tongues with a strong bone that helps them break into the juicy insides of a fruit. After they crack open a nut, they tap at the insides with their tongues.

Interestingly, they also use their tongues and beaks to explore their surroundings. They grip tree branches with their toes and also use these toes to reach for and grab fruits and nuts.

Diet

Macaws climb trees and look for fruits, nuts, flowers, and leaves. They enjoy the pulp and seeds of fruits. Some species gather at riverbanks to eat the clayey soil. They also lick at the clay on the riverbanks as it has a lot of sodium. This helps them detoxify their bodies. Along with the macaws, the parakeets, parrots, and cockatoos are also frugivorous birds.

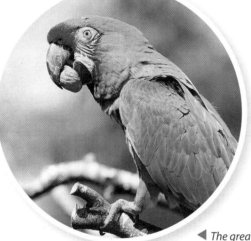

◀ *The great green macaws are 85-90 centimetres long*

Notable Macaws

The hyacinth macaw is the largest parrot and is found in Brazil, Paraguay, and Bolivia. It has a length of 100 centimetres on an average. The scarlet macaw is most famous among macaws. While the hyacinth macaw has a cobalt-blue plumage, the scarlet macaw has yellow, blue, and red plumage. Its white head easily displays that it is excited and blushing. Though they have a reputation for being difficult, macaws are still kept as pets by people around the world.

▶ *Macaws typically pick a partner and stay with them for life*

In Real Life

It is not easy to keep macaws as pets. Acquiring them can be difficult and expensive. They might make many angry noises and yelps or shrieks. They might also gnaw on a person's fingers and even bite them with their strong beaks. However, if cared for properly, they can live for as long as 100 years.

▶ *Hyacinth macaws can live up to 80 years*

The Hummingbird's Nectar

It is not just bees that hover near flowers for nectar. They get plenty of competition from birds who feed on nectar. These birds usually have thin, long beaks that they can push into the inside of a flower. One such example is the hummingbird.

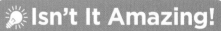

▲ Hummingbirds are the only birds than can hover in place. They do this by flapping their wings 20-80 times a second, and can move in any direction

🐾 Pollination and Diet

Hummingbirds repeatedly and quickly move their wings so that they can hover in mid-air. This way they use their beaks to feed on the sap, flowers, and nectar in the plants that they hover near. As they feed on nectar, they move from flower to flower and pollinate them. For some flowers, they might be the only source of pollination.

Hummingbirds might also feed on insects and spiders as they need to eat about two times their body weight in food. They need to do this to have enough energy to rapidly beat their wings. The rapid beating of their wings leads to a hum, which is why these birds are called hummingbirds.

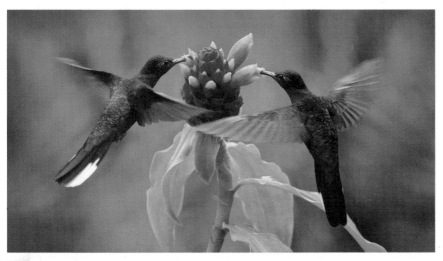

▲ The violet sabrewing is the largest species of hummingbird in Middle America

💡 Isn't It Amazing!

Usually, there are one or two collective nouns used for a group of animals. The hummingbird is unique as there are many collective nouns used to describe a group of these beautiful birds. You can call them a 'hover', 'shimmer', 'tune', or even 'bouquet'. Commonly, a group of hummingbirds is called a 'charm'. In the Caribbean, people call the hummingbird 'el zunzun'.

⭐ Incredible Individuals

John Gould (1804–1881) was a British ornithologist who named several species of hummingbirds based on their exotic appearances. He called them names like sun, sapphire, wood star, fairy, and coquette according to the colour of their feathers.

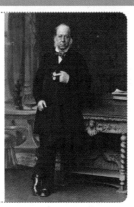

🐾 Anna's Hummingbird

The Anna's hummingbirds are unusual in that their normal body temperature is around 41° C. If their surrounding temperature falls, these hummingbirds experience a slower heart rate and as a result, their body temperature drops to nearly 8° C. They become active again once they reach their normal body temperature.

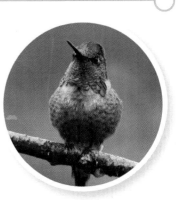

▲ Anna's hummingbird was named after Anna Masséna, the Duchess of Rivoli

Colourful Feathers

A unique feature of birds is their ability to fly. It is enabled by feathers and wings. Most birds have bright and colourful feathers with striking patterns. Besides flying, they use their feathers to keep warm in winters, keep cool in summers, camouflage themselves from predators, and attract mates.

Inside Feathers

Feathers are made of a fibrous structural protein called keratin. Each feather consists of a hollow shaft and two vanes or two halves on either side. The vanes are made up of hundreds of thin branch-like barbs. On both sides of each barb, there could be still smaller branches called barbules.

▲ *The flight feathers of the hawk help it take turns while catching prey*

A Variety of Feathers

Feathers are roughly divided into six types—contour, flight, down, filoplume, semiplume, and bristle.

01 Contour

Contour feathers are those which cover the entire body surface and give a smooth and colourful appearance. They are waterproof and protect the bird from heavy wind and hot temperatures. These contour feathers provide the streamlined structure that allows birds to fly. Contour feathers can be seen on the wings and tail of the bird where they grow from follicles present on the bird's skin.

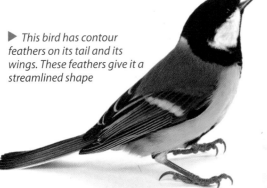

▶ *This bird has contour feathers on its tail and its wings. These feathers give it a streamlined shape*

Hollow shaft

Vane

Afterfeather

In Real Life

Nearly once every year, a bird will shed its contour feathers. These feathers will be replaced eventually. The process takes place after the breeding season is over. Even before the breeding season begins, some birds will shed some part of their contour feathers, which will then be replaced. This usually happens during the first winter of the season. This process is called 'moulting' in birds.

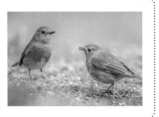

▶ *Adult robins moult at the end of the mating season*

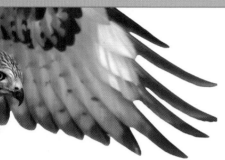

Rachis

Barb

02 Flight

Flight feathers are found in the wings and tails of birds. Of these, the flight feathers near the birds' bodies are called tertiaries. The flight feathers at the tail end are called retrices. Normally, birds have 12 tail feathers that they use to stop or make turns during flight. At the base of all flight feathers there are much smaller contour feathers called coverts which cover the wings and ears.

03 Down

Down feathers are under the contour ones and keep the birds insulated. When chicks are born, they are covered with down feathers to keep warm, but as they grow and get ready for the world, these are replaced by contour feathers to aid flight.

▼ Down feathers have a fluffy appearance as their barbs are not joined together

04 Filoplume

Filoplumes are the long, thin, and hair-like feathers with few barbs at the ends. Their function is still under debate, but they are thought to be sensory in nature. Some scientists believe that they help adjust the position of other feathers in response to air pressure.

05 Semiplume

The semiplumes shape and insulate the bird and are also useful for aerodynamics. They have long shafts and downy tips.

06 Bristle

Bristle feathers protect the birds but also act as their sensory organs. These might not be present in all birds. An insect-eating bird might have bristle feathers near the head or neck.

Bristle feathers are present near the eyelids and beak. They might be funnels that aid insect-eating birds in catching their food. These birds need to scoop insects from the earth, which bristle feathers help them do. Woodpeckers, for example, have bristle feathers near their nostrils where they act as a filter to aid the bird while it pecks at a tree.

▶ Many insect-eating birds need bristle feathers for feeding

🐾 Shed Me!

Birds shed feathers and replace them with new ones. This process is called moulting. It helps keep the feathers in good condition as it replaces the damaged and worn-out ones. Moulting is a time- and energy-consuming process. Hence, birds usually moult when they are not nesting or migrating.

How regularly do birds moult? Do they shed all their feathers at once? Some birds like eagles moult gradually and over a period of time so that they do not lose all their feathers at a time, and are capable of flying. On the other hand, birds like ducks lose their flight feathers immediately after the nesting season. During the few weeks it takes for the feathers to grow back, they remain flightless. But they do not go hungry since they find food by walking or swimming.

💡 Isn't It Amazing!

Can you imagine rubbing ants all over your body? It would hurt your skin! But birds like crows like to go 'anting' during moulting. It means to pick up ants with their beaks and rub them on their feathers and skin. The birds may also lie near anthills to allow the insects to crawl all over them. They do this because secretions from the ants soothe their irritated skin during moulting.

Play of Pigments

Feathers get their colours either due to pigments or because of light refraction caused due to the shape of the feather. Pigments are naturally colouring substances in plants, birds, and animals. In birds, pigments come in three varieties called melanin, carotenoids, and porphyrins.

Melanin

Melanin is found in both the skin and feathers of a bird. It produces colours such as black, brown, and yellow. Melanin is also known to make feathers strong and resistant. It is the primary pigment in birds such as crows, owls, and hawks.

◀ *Birds use colours to identify others of their species.*

▲ *Flamingos are born with grey feathers that slowly turn pink because of carotenoids*

Carotenoids

Birds cannot produce carotenoids but they acquire them from the food they eat. These pigments produce colours such as bright red, orange, and yellow. The flamingo looks pink, but it will lose its colour if it does not eat carotenoid-rich foods like shrimp and algae. Goldfinches and cardinals also need carotenoids.

Researchers say that there might be benefits to human consumption of carotenoids. It might reduce the risk of eye diseases and even some types of cancers. Beta-carotene is a carotenoid that is found in carrots. It can be converted into vitamin A which is beneficial for the eyes. Some carotenoids even absorb blue light that enters the eye from screens of the gadgets that we use.

In Real Life

Have you seen a bird preening? It refers to the process of cleaning and tidying the feathers. A bird preens to make sure the feathers work properly. For this, it squeezes out oil from the oil gland under its tail. With the help of the beak and claws it rubs this oil along the length of the feathers. The feathers become shiny, smooth, and waterproof.

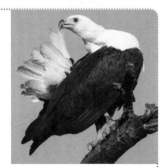

▲ *When resting, birds may preen at least once an hour*

Porphyrins

Porphyrins are pigments that can produce pink, green, and brown colours in birds. Some species of hummingbirds and peacocks get their shimmering colours from this pigment and the structure of their feathers. The colours are produced because of light refracted by the protein in the feather. The colours might vary depending on the angle at which the feather is viewed.

◀ *The Guinea turaco has a green plumage because of porphyrins*

Hide Me, See Me

Camouflage is used to conceal or blend oneself with the surroundings for safety. Birds camouflage to protect themselves as well as their eggs and later the young ones from predators. Colourful feathers are the best tools for disguise; the white-tailed ptarmigan is a great example of the same. In winter, the feathers of this bird—that resides in high altitudes—turn snow-white to blend in with the snow. In summer, the bird is streaked grey and brown. However, its tail remains white throughout the year.

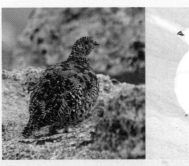

▲ *A white-tailed ptarmigan is also referred to as snow quail*

Attracting a Mate

Birds also use their feathers to attract mates, as done by the peacocks. During mating season, the male peacock spreads out its beautiful blue and green tail and puts on an elaborate show to attract the peahen, a regular-looking, brown bird. Flamingos, the beautiful pink birds, rub themselves with carotenoid-rich oil from their tail glands to look pinker and more desirable to their mates.

▼ *Peacocks take three years to grow their tail feathers*

The Wonder of Wings

Do you ever wonder how or why wings evolved? One theory states that forelimbs were modified into wings. According to another theory, wings were used as display objects to attract mates, while still another says wings evolved from gliding ancestors. Whichever the theory, birds could not have taken flight without these structures.

▲ *The huge wings of eagles help them soar and glide with minimal effort*

Is it a Bird? Is it a Plane?

The wings of an aeroplane are modelled on bird wings. Wings are attached to powerful chest muscles. They are convex on the upper surface, concave on the lower, and they taper from front to back.

When a bird flies, air flows at greater speed at the upper part of the wing than the lower part because of its shape, creating less pressure on the top. This helps lift the bird during flight.

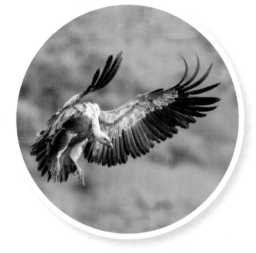

How Birds Use Wings

There are different types of wings based on the flight of the bird. Birds of prey like eagles, vultures, and hawks have soaring wings that are large and broad. The moment the bird spots prey, it closes its wings and dives down, opening them again to slow down as it nears the ground to make a soft landing.

◀ *A Cape vulture has a wingspan of 2.26–2.6 metres*

▶ *Adult European gulls have white heads and bodies and grey wings*

Birds such as seagulls and Arctic terns have gliding wings. These are long, narrow, and flat, with no space between the feathers. Gliding wings allow the birds to fly without having to spend much energy to stay in the air. Gliding refers to a bird moving in a downward direction closer to land and thus it must occasionally flap its wings to regain height.

Small birds such as house sparrows, woodpeckers, and thrushes must be quick to escape their predators. They have elliptical wings. These rapid take-off wings have spaces between the feathers, making them lighter and easier to move. These wings are not made for sustained flight and the birds must expend a lot of energy to stay airborne for long periods of time. Scavenger birds such as crows and ravens also have elliptical wings that help them steal food and escape quickly.

◀ *The flying sparrow has high-speed wings*

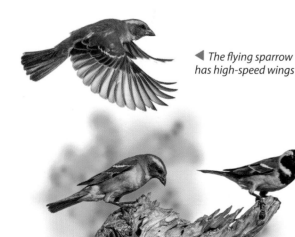

Birds such as swallows and swifts, which must catch their food mid-air at times, have high-speed wings. These wings are long, narrow, and pointed. They are angled backwards, making rapid flight easy.

The No-Fly List

It is not true that all birds fly. Even though they have wings, birds like ostriches, emus, kiwis, rheas, and cassowaries cannot fly. Their flat breastbone, to which the strong flight muscles are attached, lack a keel. This means that their wings are weak and cannot take off the ground. Flightless birds as a group are called **ratites**.

Long Lost Cousins

It is believed that ratites are related to a group of 47 South American birds called 'tinamou'. While ratites lost their ability to fly over time, tinamous are capable of flight, but prefer to walk on the ground.

Scientists believe that over millions of years, ratites lost flight as a trait as they adapted to their environment. Wings became a redundant feature. However, the birds evolved strong muscular legs instead, making them fast runners and offering an alternative way to escape predators.

World's Biggest Bird

The ostrich is the largest living flightless bird. It is native to the continent of Africa. In fact, even the egg the ostrich lays is the largest of all eggs, each about 6 inches in length, 15-18 inches in circumference, and around 1.4 kilograms. When it senses danger, the bird shoots off at a speed of 72 kmph and while facing a threat, it is known to kick hard.

The Australian Wonder

The emu is the second-largest living bird in the world. It is about 5 feet tall and is found on the continent of Australia. Like the ostrich it runs very fast, at 48 kmph, and kicks at the predator.

South American Rhea

Rheas are found in South America. They are omnivores, which means that they eat both plants and animals. They are related to the ostrich and emu—who live in different continents. But, they are much smaller, measuring 4 feet in height and 20 kilograms in weight.

Rheas are of two types—the common rhea which is found in Brazil and Argentina, and its cousin, which is a slightly smaller bird called Darwin's rhea, which lives in areas starting from Peru, all the way down to Patagonia.

Isn't It Amazing!

When dinosaurs were wiped off the planet, mammals were still small and had not yet evolved to become apex predators. Instead, birds underwent what is known as an 'evolutionary explosion'—occupying several ecological niches. Some, like the hummingbird, evolved to be very tiny and live on nectar, while others like the giant moa became large herbivores. Birds were successful because they could fly and take off at will, successfully defending themselves from enemies. They were also able to reach farther than mammals to find food and shelter.

◀ The adult ostrich is 9 ft in height

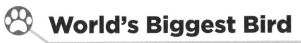

▶ Emus are the only birds with calf muscles

◀ Ostriches have two toes, but rheas have three

▼ One ostrich egg is equivalent to 24 hen's eggs

Amazing Homes

Birds build nests to lay eggs and nurture their young ones. It is a tedious task because they have no workforce, cement, bricks, and tiles. They use their beaks and feet to put a home together with basic material such as grass, twigs, leaves, mud, stones, and even small pieces of cloth. Some birds do not build nests; they dig small, shallow holes to lay eggs, while others lay eggs on open land.

Sociable Weaver

The sociable weaver bird is a species found in South Africa. These birds believe in community living. They build huge nests with individual chambers which can house more than 100 breeding pairs of birds. Nests are built with grass and can reach a height of 3 metres. One can find these nests perched on trees and poles.

Hammerhead

It is a wading bird found in Africa and Madagascar. It builds 4–5 nests a year using as many as 10,000 pieces of twigs, reeds, and grasses. It holds the nest together with mud as this provides insulation on cold nights. Both male and female birds build nests that can span 4 feet in height and weigh up to 50 kilograms.

European Bee-eater

The European bee-eater is a small bird found in southern Europe and parts of Africa and Asia. The bird nests in a hole in the riverbanks sand. It drills the hole with its beak and then clears the sand with its feet, making a small burrow. It is a smart bird, as it makes sure the soil is soft enough to drill a hole, but also safe enough to prevent caving in.

Swiftlet

The swiftlet is a small bird dwelling in South East Asia. The unique thing about this bird is that it builds its nest with its own saliva. The nest is built in layers, usually on walls of caves, buildings, or against cliffs. The birds live in huge colonies. The nest is used in a delicacy called the bird's-nest soup in Chinese cuisine.

Common Murres

The common murres are medium-sized water birds. These are commonly seen on the Pacific Coast in places such as Alaska and Canada, near bays and the ocean. These birds nest on open ledges on rock cliffs. Their nests are huge, packed colonies. Since the eggs are in the open, one of the parents stands guard to protect it from predators.

Cuckoo

Cuckoos do not build their own nests, instead, they let other birds do all the work. They lay eggs in magpie nests. Instead of waiting for the magpies to leave the nest, research has shown that female cuckoos force the female magpies out of the nest to lay their eggs. Some cuckoo birds resemble the predatory hawk, scaring the magpie into fleeing, while the cuckoo reaches the nest without a fight. The poor female magpie then incubates these eggs along with her own.

Flamingo

Flamingos live in colonies. During the breeding season, most of these birds mate at the same time, laying eggs in smooth conical mud piles, which are their nests. The nests are built by both males and females in shallow lagoons.

Bald Eagle

Bald eagles build nests (called eyries) high up on tree branches from where they can view their surroundings and others cannot reach easily. The nest is usually close to water. Both male and female eagles build the nest with small branches, grass, and twigs. They are not just deep, but large as well, and can span as much as 5 feet wide.

Migrating Birds

Migration is a periodic, seasonal movement of animals from one place to another. It is particularly evident in birds. Most often, birds leave a place in autumn and return to it in spring. To avoid harsh winters they move to a place with plenty of sunshine and food. Migration and breeding are both required for survival of the different species of birds.

Path Taken

Migrating birds take the same route every year and usually it is the direct path between two places. This is done to conserve energy. It is said that for navigation they depend on the movement of the Sun and Earth's magnetic field. Hills, mountains, forests, rivers and coastlines act as guides during the trip.

Some species of birds use the night skies to fly to their destination. The orientation of the stars helps them steer in the right direction. Birds usually migrate in flocks and many use the V-shaped formation while flying to conserve their energy.

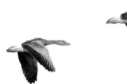
▶ About 40 per cent of birds all over the world migrate regularly

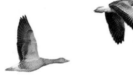

▼ Robins are fiercely territorial over food supply

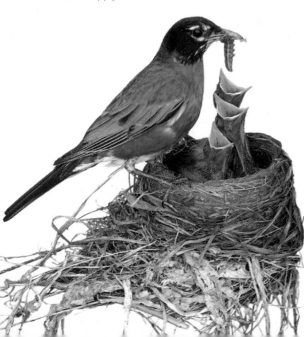

A Dangerous Journey

During migration, birds face many hazards in the form of storms, predators, and at times disorientation, especially while crossing deserts or large water bodies like seas and oceans. Added to this list are the dangers they face from human activity like habitat loss because of deforestation, skyscrapers, cell phone towers, television towers, and electric cables.

Little Birdies

Apart from survival, birds have another purpose for migration. In spring, when the weather is good, there is plenty of food and foliage to hide their eggs and keep young ones safe. Birds return to their breeding grounds to procreate. However, there is one bird which returns to its nesting ground in winter to lay eggs. It is the emperor penguin!

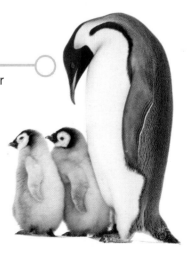
▶ Emperor penguins are the tallest and heaviest of all penguin species

In Real Life

Siberian cranes are an **endangered species**. Every year, the birds migrate from their habitats in Central Asia to reach India during the winter season. However, in the past few years, none of these migrating birds have been spotted in India, especially in Bharatpur, Rajasthan, which was famous for their sightings. This might be due to ecological damage to their habitat and hunting of these beautiful birds for their meat.

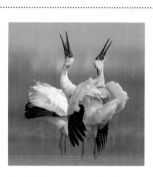

▲ Siberian cranes feed on roots and berries

▲ Red grouse are ground-dwelling birds, but they can also fly short distances and perform twists and turns in the air

◀ Migratory route of the Arctic tern. They have the longest annual migration of any animal on Earth

▲ Arctic terns migrate to and from the Arctic Circle and the Antarctic Circle

Arctic Tern

This small bird breeds in summer in the Arctic. In the autumn it is ready to fly south to Antarctica. After spending about three months there, it flies back once more to Greenland or Canada where it dwells. The bird is special because it travels the longest migratory distance of any animal on this planet. It covers a total of about 96,000 kilometres in a roundabout trip.

Sedentary Birds

Some birds like the Siberian crane and Eurasian cuckoo are known to migrate thousands of kilometres, while others such as the American robin travel short distances. Some birds like the red grouse found in Great Britain do not migrate at all. Such birds are called sedentary or resident birds.

Sedentary birds do not migrate because they find food all year long in places where they reside. Few birds such as the skylarks and snow buntings migrate from their homes in higher altitudes to lower altitudes in winters.

Isn't It Amazing!

Lesser flamingos live in the Rift Valley of Africa and feed on algal blooms found in the lakes in the area. These blooms could be toxic to many, but lesser flamingos thrive on them. The interesting fact is that the birds are not migratory, but nomadic, moving from one lake to another in search of ample food.

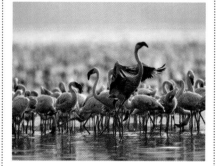

▲ Flamingos can filter feed in water for several hours a day

Breeding Season

For the emperor penguin, the breeding season usually starts in April. This is autumn in Antarctica. The sea ice, which might have melted in summer, is in the process of refreezing. Emperor penguins are the only animals which breed in the Antarctic winter. The birds make no nests. As a matter of fact, it is the male that cares for the young ones, while the female goes out in search of food.

02 May–June

Come May or early June, it is time for the female to leave the colony in search of food. She gives the egg for incubation to the male. The male pushes the egg between its feet, under a feathered skinfold called the brood pouch. The egg stays warm and snug at 38° C, even though the temperature outside is way below 0° C.

The maintenance of temperature is very important as an exposed egg could freeze in the surrounding temperatures, killing the embryo inside. It is a tough road for the papa penguin!

03 July–August

The colony becomes quiet when the females leave in search of food. They return in July. They trudge through the snow and blizzards. The trek to the sea can be 80 km at times. The females feed themselves on foods like fish, krill, and squid.

▲ *A female gentoo penguin trekking to the water*

01 April

Emperor penguins can be seen in thousands. It is freezing cold. The temperatures are close to 60° C with wind speeds of almost 200 kmph. But, it is time to procreate and hence time to find a mate. There is a lot of hustle and bustle in the colony as the penguins go looking for mates. They sing songs, march in an impressive manner or bow their heads together. Once they find their partner, they mate. The female produces a single egg.

▲ *The male penguin incubates the egg*

▲ *The male and female emperor during the mating season*

👥 In Real Life

Research has found that emperor penguins breed on ice shelves. While some breeds live on sea-ice, some are also found to live on the ice shelves. As they rely on the ice, the population of emperor penguins could rapidly decline due to global warming.

04 July-August

By the time the females return, the male penguins are famished. They have not eaten anything for more than two months. Their only source of energy is their body fat. They have lost more than half their body weight. On the other hand, the females are big and well-fed. After their return, the female and male find each other using calls. She **regurgitates** some food and feeds the male penguin. The male gives the egg, or if it has hatched, the chick, to the female and begins its journey to the sea to find food. But at times the male is adamant on not giving the egg to the female. He has looked after it for so many months after all. The female has to really work hard to convince the male to give up the egg, so that he can go search for food.

▲ A gentoo female penguin feeding its chicks

💡 Isn't It Amazing!

It might surprise people to learn that there are penguins in Africa! The African penguins, like the emperor penguin, have black and white feathers. These feathers keep them warm and dry in their home on the coastlines of Africa. These penguins belong to one of the smallest species.

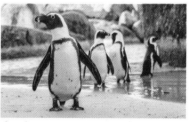

▲ African penguins are also called 'jackass' penguins

◀ A crèche of emperor penguins

05 September

By September, the chicks grow up. They can keep themselves insulated. They need a lot more food to grow even further. The young emperor penguin needs both the parents (males are back in the colony by this time) to look for food. The parent emperor penguins leave the young in groups called 'crèches' and go hunting for food.

06 December

By December, the summer sets in the Southern Hemisphere. The ice breaks, bringing the nesting site close to the sea water. The chicks grow up into young adults. They are now capable of swimming and finding food on their own.

▲ An Adélie penguin jumping between ice floes

Knowing Birds

Did you know that there are people in the world who have dedicated their lives to learning about birds? In fact, it is an entire field of study on its own! The branch of science which deals with the study of birds is called **ornithology** and the person who studies birds is called an **ornithologist**.

Ornithology

The basic equipment any ornithologist needs is a good pair of binoculars to observe the birds. These professionals study the day-to-day lives of birds, including their feeding habits, flying techniques, mating and nesting patterns, as well as migrations. Some famous ornithologists from around the world are Allan Octavian Hume, Dr Salim Ali, Peter Scott, and Roger Tory Peterson. Read on to know some special habits and traits of birds.

★ Incredible Individuals

Dr Salim Ali (1896–1987) was called the 'birdman of India' because of his contributions to the field of ornithology.

The Himalayan forest thrush, which was discovered by a group of Indian and Swedish scientists, was given the scientific name *Zoothera salimalii* in honour of Dr Salim Ali.

Bird Brain

To be bird-brained means to be stupid, as birds are supposed to have small brains. Are birds really dumb though? No! Scientists have proven that birds have lots of neurons in their brains, meaning that they are intelligent. Firstly, birds migrate with an accurate sense of direction, so much so that they come back to the same homing ground they left before migration.

Studies have proven that ravens plan tasks in advance like humans; crows remember faces; parrots, especially the African grey parrot, can mimic human speech; and cockatoos, among other birds, can create music. While courting a female, a male cockatoo can create its own music by beating seed pods and twigs against tree hollows.

The Intelligent Owl

The barn owl cannot see well, but its sense of hearing is very keen. It can hear well enough to locate its prey, usually a mouse or shrew, even in thick grass. The two ears of the owl are different from each other. Its left ear can detect sounds from below, while the right can hear sounds above it. Also, the barn owl has thick and soft feathers, which make minimum noise, so the prey is not alerted.

◀ *Barn owls are amongst the most intelligent birds and have a sharp sense of hearing*

▼ *Ornithologists had a vital role to play in the protection of birds, especially from commercial hunting for food and millinery trade*

👤 In Real Life

Birds are an important part of cultures around the world. In the *Bible*, Noah is said to have sent out a dove to see if the flood waters on Earth had receded. In India, spotting of the crow pheasant is considered a good omen, while in China the crane is a symbol of peace and longevity.

Cause and Effect

Humans do not realise it, but birds are not just things of beauty that soar in our skies. They help us in many ways. They fertilise plants, disperse seeds, help in pollination, clean up carrion, and control the populations of various insects. Today, more than 12 per cent of bird species are endangered.

In Africa, the population of eagles and vultures is dipping, while migratory birds such as the spoonbills, pelicans, and storks near the Yellow Sea are endangered. Penguins are facing a threat to their existence as the ice cover decreases in Antarctica.

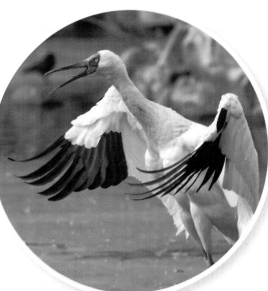

▲ No sightings of Siberian cranes have been reported at Bharatpur, Rajasthan in recent years and only 3,200 remain in the world

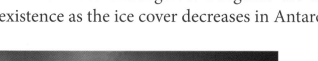

▲ Animals and birds are losing their homes due to deforestation

Reasons for Extinction

The presence of harmful chemicals such as DDT in the atmosphere is one of the main reasons that birds face extinction. Although DDT has been banned since the 1970s (except in some malaria-prone areas of Africa), its harmful **hereditary** effects are still felt by many birds of prey in the USA. Other causes for extinction are air and marine pollution, hunting, deforestation, development in and around ecological habitats, and climate and weather changes.

International Union for Conservation of Nature

International Union for Conservation of Nature (IUCN) is an organisation established in 1948 which works towards conservation and sustainability of the environment. The IUCN Red List of Threatened Species, established in 1964, is one of the world's most reliable sources of information on global conservation of animals, plants, and fungi.

The organisation has created varied categories based on the risks faced by animals, birds, and fungi. The animals for whom the organisation has sufficient data are divided into the following categories:

● Extinct (EX) ● Extinct in Wild (EW) ● Critically Endangered (CR) ● Endangered (EN)

● Vulnerable (VU) ● Near Threatened (NT) ● Least Concern (LC)

Do Your Bit

The government will do its bit but is there something you can do to help? You can help by educating people and creating awareness about our environment. Further, we must all strive hard to protect the trees, as they are homes, not just to the birds, but to many insects and smaller animals as well. See if you can join a good conservation programme with the help of a family member.

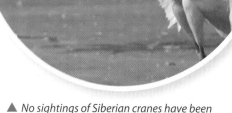

Planting trees will create more homes for birds

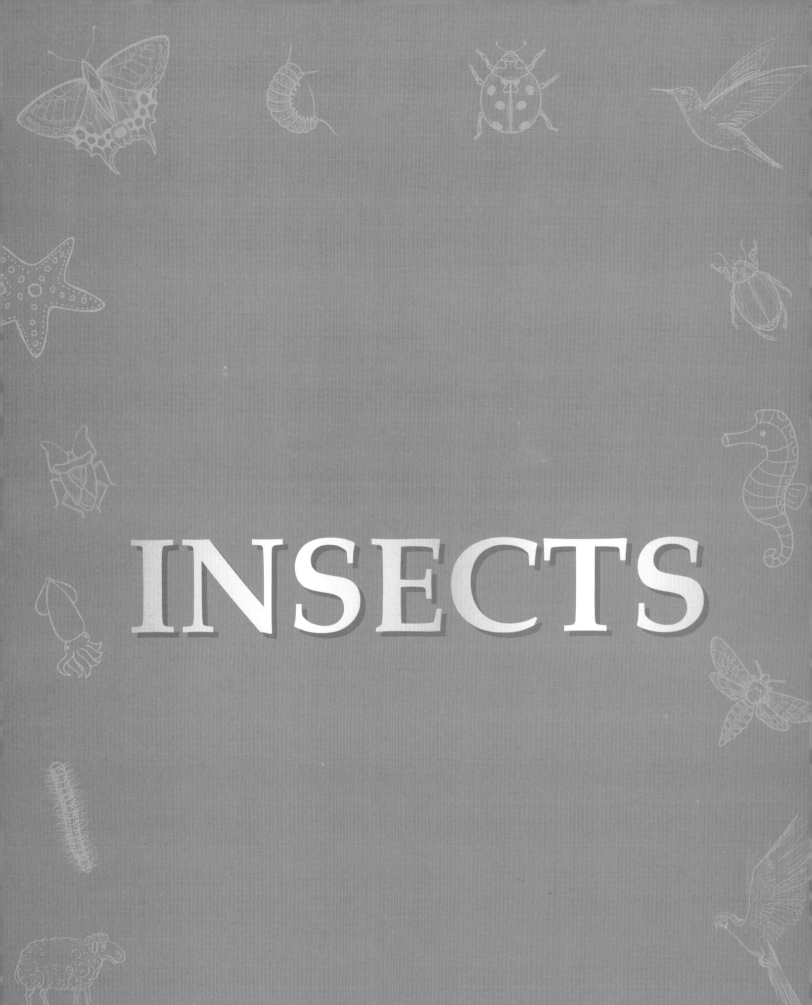

INSECTS

CREEPY CRAWLIES

Think about all the insects that you see around you. Did you know that some are only found in tropical forests? There also exist poisonous insects, insects that have six legs, and even insects that can fly. Around a million insect species have already been discovered, but scientists estimate that there might be many many more out there. Insects are extremely varied and exist in large numbers. It is estimated that for every human on the planet, we have 1.4 billion insects to match.

They are a group so diverse and widely spread out that they cover all the nooks and crevices of the world, from the Arctic snow to desert rocks, and from deep oceans to hot springs. In fact, a single swarm of desert locusts can cover an area of 1,200 square kilometres and contains close to 80 million insects. No wonder they are a part of our daily lives. Read on to learn about the interesting world of insects.

▼ *The butterfly too is an insect. It transforms from a caterpillar and sprouts those colourful wings*

Spot the Insect

Insects account for almost 80 per cent of the animal species in the world. Now that is a huge number! All of these insects belong to the larger group of invertebrate animals known as **arthropods**. This is the same group to which scorpions, spiders, crabs, and lobsters belong.

Body

An adult insect found anywhere in the world has three common body parts—head, thorax, and abdomen. Most insects have three pairs of legs, two pairs of wings, and two antennae. The eyes, mouth, and antennae are on the head; the legs and wings are attached to the thorax. The abdomen has most of the organs, such as the stomach and intestine.

▼ *The jewel beetle is one of the most colourful insects in the world, belonging to order Coleoptera*

Exoskeleton

Insects are covered with a hard exoskeleton made up of chitin, which contains proteins and carbohydrates. In an insect, the eyes are covered with a thin layer of exoskeleton. This is a non-living structure; hence it does not grow with the insect. At every stage of growth, the insect moults.

Moulting refers to the process by which the exoskeleton is shed to regrow a new one. At this point of time the insect, with its soft exterior, is most vulnerable to predators and its surrounding environment. Many insects go into hiding until the tough, new exoskeleton grows back.

Apart from protection, the exoskeleton of the insect gives its body shape and prevents it from drying. It has tiny holes called **spiracles**. These are small openings or pores that allow respiration. The exoskeleton is made up of varied patterns and colours. Bright colours warn the predators that the insect is poisonous, while dull colours make for good camouflage.

◀ *A cicada shedding its exoskeleton while entering the next stage of its life*

Classification

All insects belong to the class Insecta. They are classified into several groups. Most of the insects on our planet belong to the following orders—Coleoptera (scarabs and beetles), Lepidoptera (butterflies and moths), Hymenoptera (ants, wasps, and bees), and Diptera (flies or 'true' flies).

There are many species of insects belonging to each of these classes. 40 per cent of the known species of insects belong to order Coleoptera. The order Lepidoptera has about 180,000 species of insects. Order Hymenoptera has about 115,000 known species, while around 125,000 species belong to order Diptera.

Sense-able

Insects have a good sense of touch, smell, hearing, and sight. They do not have ears, but their skin can pick up sound waves. For a few insects such as grasshoppers and crickets, the tympanal organ acts like the ears. Insects use their antennae to feel and smell. They need to have a keen sense of smell to detect food and mates.

Eyesight

Insect eyes can detect movement but cannot see shapes as we do. Not all insects can see colours, but few, such as butterflies have exceptional vision to find flowers.

Insects can have two types of eyes; each species might have either of the types or both. The first type are called the ocelli. These are simple, small eyes. They cannot see well but can detect dark and light. These eyes are seen on insects like fleas.

The second type are huge, bulging eyes like that of the housefly. These are called compound eyes. They are made up of many tiny single eyes. Each single eye is called the ommatidium. It sees its own image and sends it to the insect brain. The brain then combines all the images to form a bigger picture.

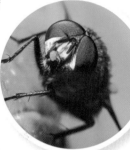

▲ *Wasps and ants have both types of eyes*

Of Legs and Joints

The word 'arthropod' means to have jointed feet. Insects are arthropods, which means their legs have joints just like the joints on human legs. However, their legs do not have bones inside them; they have muscles instead. These muscles allow the insects to move, bend, run, and jump.

One of the fastest insects in the world is the Australian tiger beetle. It cannot fly but can run at a speed of 9 kmph. Another fast insect is the tiger moth caterpillar which picks up a speed of 5 kmph.

Wings

Insect wings are made up of chitin. The muscles attached to the exoskeleton make these wings flap. Most insects such as bees, beetles, and dragonflies have two pairs. Insect wings are thin and transparent, but veins running between them make them sturdy.

▲ *A species of grasshopper called tropidacris cristata*

This is not to say that all insects have wings. Remember, there is great diversity in the insect world. Fleas, lice, and bedbugs, for example, are wingless. Few insects such as aphids can even grow wings whenever needed, such as in the case of food shortage or overcrowding. At such times, the insects need wings to fly away to a better place. Aphids are commonly called greenflies and blackflies. Many aphid species choose to feed on only one type of plant for their entire lives. So, they are called **monophagous**.

Isn't It Amazing!

Cicadas are among the loudest insects in the world. They have special organs called tymbals that produce their characteristic sounds which can sometimes reach 90 decibels! This is as loud as the sound produced by a motorcycle.

The Menacing Weevil

Beetles and weevils belong to the order Coleoptera. This order has close to 350,000 insect species. Coleoptera is not just the largest insect order, but also the largest group of animals in the world. The number of insects classified within this order is rising each year with the discovery of new species by scientists. Coleopterans are seen in almost all habitats of the world, right from oceans, mountains, and deserts to cold regions.

🐾 Colourful Beetles

The word 'Coleoptera' comes from the Greek words, '*koleos*' or sheath and '*pteron*' or wings. This refers to the special arrangements of wings in beetles. Similar to other insects, beetles have two pairs of wings. However, one pair is slightly modified.

The front wings in these beetles are hard and strong. They cover the upper side of the body like a sheath. This hard casing-like structure is called the **elytra**. Elytra protect the delicate rear wings. The rear wings are folded under the elytra at rest, but when the beetle is about to fly, they emerge from the casing.

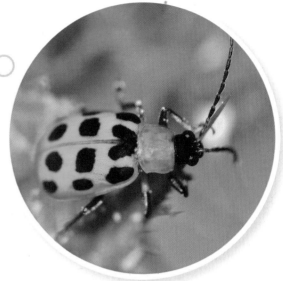

▲ *Beetles exist in different colours. This is the spotted cucumber beetle*

🐾 Weevils

There are about 40,000 species of weevils in existence in the world. Most species are brown or grey, but the diamond beetle is colourful. Weevils are also called snout beetles because they have long, curved snouts which look like elephant trunks. The snouts are used to make holes in leaves to lay eggs. They are also used to penetrate the leaves.

Most weevils have long foldable antennae. These antennae fold into special grooves present on the snout. They are small animals, measuring about 6 millimetres; but there are exceptions with few measuring almost up to 7–8 centimetres. Weevils feed on fruits, stems, flowers, and seeds.

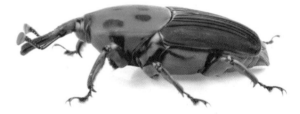

▲ *Weevils have managed to survive because of their snouts*

🐾 Into the Grain

Grain weevils are small brown weevils, not more than 4 millimetres long. They make the most menacing pests as they destroy stored grain such as maize, oats, and wheat. The females bore holes in individual grains to lay eggs. The larvae, which emerge from these eggs, feed on the grain. When they are threatened, they feign death. This is how they protect themselves from predators.

🐾 Cotton Soft

The boll weevil is about 6 millimetres in length. But it makes for a terrible guest, as it enjoys destroying its host—the cotton bolls. The female boll weevil lays eggs in cotton buds. The larvae from the eggs feed on the cotton seeds as well as fibres, completely destroying them. Farmers have to bear immense losses every year because of the boll weevils.

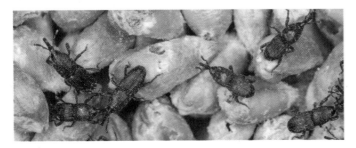

▲ *Grain weevils are also known as wheat weevils*

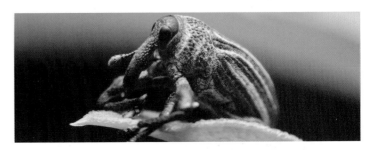

▲ *Boll weevils cannot feed or breed on any plant other than cotton*

The Colourful Scarab

Scarabs are a big family of beetles comprising more than 30,000 species. That means that 10 per cent of all known beetles are actually scarabs! The sacred scarab is one of the most famous members of the scarab family. In ancient Egypt, it was worshipped as the incarnation of the Sun god Khepri. Various species of scarabs are found all around the world, except for Antarctica and the oceans.

Appearance

Scarabs are usually black or brown in colour, but there exist species which are mesmerising with bright colours, beautiful patterns, and metallic sheens. They are oval in shape with stout bodies. Sizes could vary with the smallest being just about 2 millimetres and the largest being around 17 centimetres.

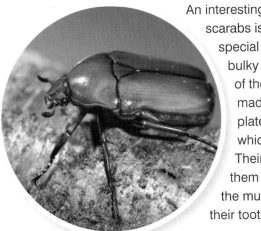

An interesting feature of the scarabs is the presence of special antennae on their bulky bodies. The ends of the antennae are made up of three flat plate-like structures which form a club. Their front legs allow them to freely dig in the mud because of their toothed edges.

▲ Rings made of scarab beetles were military symbols in ancient Rome

▲ This insect with a seemingly metallic sheen belongs to a species of beetle called Protaetia

Diet

Scarabs have a varied diet. Some species eat fruits, insects, as well as carrion, while others eat the slime of snails. Some, like the Japanese beetles, are pests. Did you know that a large group of Japanese beetles can eat the leaves and fruits of a peach tree within a few minutes, leaving only the branches behind?

Incredible Individuals

In Egyptian mythology, all the main gods acquired the characteristics of creator gods. A single figure could have many names; among those of the Sun god, the most important were Khepri (the morning form), Re-Harakhty (a form of Re associated with Horus), and Atum (the old, evening form). Khepri was associated with the scarab beetle because the ancient Egyptians associated the insect rolling a ball of dung on the floor with the invisible forces that contributed to the movements of the Sun in the sky.

Dung Beetles

Dung beetles come in varieties called rollers, tunnellers, and dwellers, depending upon how they treat the dung. Rollers simply make dung balls which they roll away and store in a safe place to consume later or use the balls to lay eggs. On the other hand, the dwellers use the dung as their home. Females lay their eggs in the dung and when the larvae emerge, they have food to eat. The tunnellers create a tunnel underneath the waste material.

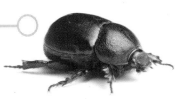

▲ Dung beetles can roll up to 1,141 times their weight, which is why they are the strongest insect in the world

The Helpful Ladybug

The ladybug is a small, beautiful insect with a shiny red and black body bearing seven black spots. There are 5,000 species of these insects, but the red-and-black spotted ladybug is the most famous. Ladybugs belong to the beetle family. They are also known as ladybirds or lady beetles. Read on to find out how the insect got this interesting name.

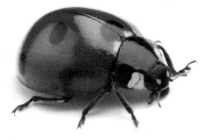

▲ The spots on ladybugs are meant to warn attackers that these beetles taste terrible

▲ Ladybugs pose no threat to human beings

🐾 Behaviour

Ladybugs are found in varied habitats. They live in forests, grasslands, cities, and even on farms. In cold weather they **hibernate** in rocks, farm homes, or logs.

These tiny creatures are oval with a dome-shaped structure on their backs and tiny legs. They come in various colours such as red, orange, yellow, black, and pink. These colours serve as a warning to the predators. If ladybugs feel threatened, they release a foul-smelling liquid from the joints in their legs. They are also known to play dead at times in the presence of a predator. Adult females lay eggs near insect colonies. Once the larvae emerge, the first thing they do is eat. The form and behaviour of beetles, even the ladybugs, have inspired many inventions among people. The car manufacturer Volkswagen created a car inspired by and named after beetles.

🐾 A Holy Name

Ladybugs are not just good to look at; they are also very useful to farmers as they devour aphids and other insects which can harm their crops. A single ladybug can eat close to 5,000 insects in its lifetime. That is a lot for such a small creature.

Long ago in Europe, farmers were being harassed by crop-eating insects. They began to pray to the Virgin Mary for help. Then they realised that there was one insect which helped them eat up these pests; it was the ladybug. As a thanks to the Virgin Mary for saving their crops, they called the insect 'beetle of our Lady'. As the years passed, the name changed to ladybug. However, not all ladybugs are nice to crops. The Mexican bean beetle, a species of the ladybug, eats the bean plant, while the squash beetle eats the squash plant.

▲ A Mexican bean beetle prefers the beans growing on a bean plant as its host

👤 In Real Life

Beetles hate salt water. But some species love fresh water. The diving beetles use their hairy legs as oars to wade in the water. Of course, they have to come to the surface every few minutes to gulp in air. The Namib Desert beetle is a species that lives in the deserts of Africa, where water is sparse. It survives in the desert by harvesting moisture from the air, condensing it on its back and storing the water. This has inspired human beings to conserve water using innovative techniques.

The Glowing Firefly

Fireflies can glow. On hot summer nights, if you step outside, especially where there is quiet and peace, you might find a mild, intermittent glow coming from some trees. Deep in the forests these glows are aplenty. The source is the firefly, a type of beetle. There are about 2,000 known species of fireflies in the world.

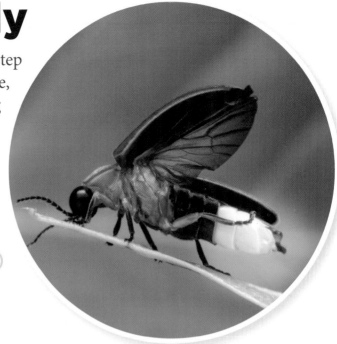

▲ *The light shows of fireflies are mating acts*

What are Fireflies?

Fireflies are soft-bodied beetles, about 2.5 centimetres long. They are black or brown in colour with yellow or orange markings. Most fireflies are nocturnal insects, but there are some species which are diurnal. That means some fireflies are active in the day and night. Adult fireflies survive on pollen and nectar, while there are also some which do not eat at all. In a few cases, the female of one species targets the male from another as prey. Fireflies love warmth, which is why they are a common occurrence in the humid regions of Asia and North America. They are found in the temperate belt near damp places.

Glow in the Dark

The glow of the fireflies comes from an organ located underneath their abdomen. In the organs are special cells which carry a substance called luciferin. The fireflies take in oxygen and combine it with luciferin to produce their characteristic glow. Scientifically, the glow is called **bioluminescence**, which means the production of light by a living organism.

The luminescence of fireflies is specific to species. Scientists still have to unravel the mystery of the intermittent glowing patterns displayed by these insects. So far, we know that the light is emitted to not just attract potential mates but also to warn a predator to keep away.

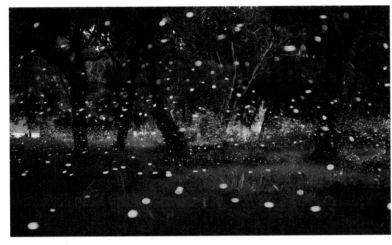

▲ *Some species of fireflies synchronize their flashing*

Glow Worms

Females lay eggs in the ground. After the incubation period, the larvae emerge from the eggs and are called glow worms. This is because even the larva of a firefly can emit a glow. The larvae live on the ground, feeding on snails, slugs, and some other types of worms. Before eating, the larvae inject a sort of numbing fluid into the prey.

Finding Fireflies

People can see fireflies in the jungles of Southeast Asia, especially Thailand, Malaysia, Philippines, China, and India. People from these places have reported seeing 'the dance of the fireflies'. In USA, the insects put up a great show at the Great Smoky Mountain National Park. Fireflies are also found in abundance in the humid rainforests of Central and South America, and parts of Australia. Remember to be quiet when you want to see their beautiful glow.

Isn't It Amazing!

The African Goliath beetle is named after the biblical giant Goliath. No wonder, because this is one of the heaviest insects in the world. It weighs close to 100 grams.

Butterfly or Moth?

Butterflies and moths belong to order Lepidoptera, whose name means 'scaly wings'. The large, thin wings of these insects are covered with tiny scales. Along with the wings, the body and legs too are covered with scales, which come off if the insects are held. The order Lepidoptera is the biggest family of insects after Coleoptera. It consists of almost 180,000 species.

Similar but Different

There is a reason that butterflies and moths look similar—they are cousins! However, they have many differences which make it easy to tell them apart. There are 20,000 species of butterflies, but there are a whopping 160,000 species of moths. While butterflies are active during the day, moths are active during the night. Butterflies sport bright and beautiful colours. But moths often have dull brown or grey patterns on their wings. Butterflies have club-like antennae, while moths have feathery antennae.

An interesting thing about these insects is that when butterflies are at rest, they hold their wings vertically in place. But moths have a variety of ways to hold their wings. They hold their wings like a tent above their bodies, or spread them out horizontally, and even wrap them around their bodies.

Sweet Nectar

What do butterflies and moths feed on? They eat the nectar produced in flowers. Nectar is a food source containing lots of energy-rich sugars. Butterflies and moths eat nectar when they become adults as they need lots of energy to fly. In tropical forests, nectar is available all year. However, in cold regions, flower production is seasonal, so butterflies and moths have a corresponding life cycle.

Butterflies and moths have a unique ability not seen in other insects. They can coil up their proboscis or feeding tube. To sip nectar from deep in the flower, the feeding tube becomes straight. It is used like a straw to suck out the sweet substance.

Apart from nectar, few species are also known to feed on mosses, lichens, ferns and even grains. The flour moth is one such insect, it devours stored grains and cereals. The fungus moth and scavenger moth feed on decaying and dead plant remains.

◀ *Butterflies actually have four wings, not two*

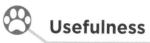

▶ *Butterflies come in various colours and patterns. Several of them hide from predators using their colourful wings*

Usefulness

Lepidopterans have made homes in all continents except Antarctica. They live in forests, grasslands, mountains, deserts, and even cities. Due to their various hues and patterns, butterflies are considered to be beautiful and are captured in art by humans. They have served as inspiration in designing jewellery and decorative ornaments as well as in the clothing industry.

Lepidopterans have been used to study the environment as well as changes in the climate. They also help the country benefit monetarily as butterfly parks and tours have been set up in many parts of the world. Tourists take these up in hordes.

Butterflies and moths are important **cross pollinators**. For example, the South American cactus moth has been introduced in Australia to clear out hectares and hectares of prickly pear cactus, a weed harmful to crops.

In Real Life

Moths are nocturnal insects. They are attracted to light because of a phenomenon called phototaxis. The movement of their wings is influenced by the strength of light. With distant sources of light, such as the Moon, the light reaches equally to both eyes, thereby causing the insect to fly in a straight line. But if the source of light is closer, such as a candle flame or electric bulb, the moth perceives it strongly in one eye rather than in both eyes. As a result, the wings on one side are stimulated to move faster, causing the insect to fly right into the light source.

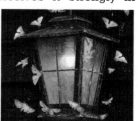

▲ *Many adult moths don't eat*

🐾 Trivia

The peacock butterfly has a special pattern on its wings that looks like eyes. It uses these eyespots to scare and ward off predators.

The purple bog fritillary is a polar insect living in cold temperatures all through the year. These butterflies have dark and hairy bodies to absorb more heat. They are smaller than the average butterfly so that they can warm up quickly.

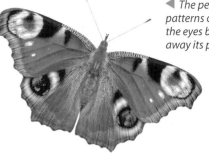

◀ *The peacock butterfly has eye-shaped patterns on its wings. It sits in a way that the eyes become prominent, scaring away its predators*

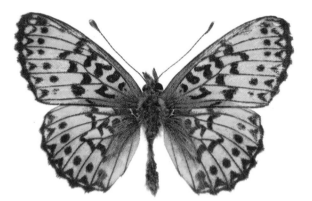

▲ *The patterns on the underside of the purple bog fritillary butterflies are lighter than their dorsal or upper side patterns*

The western spruce budworm moth mainly consumes needles of fir and spruce. But the larvae of this moth are devastating pests affecting the coniferous forests of the USA and Canada. Infestation densities as low as 15–20 caterpillars per square metre can lead to rapid **defoliation** and further death of the trees.

The sunset moth found in Madagascar is often mistaken for a butterfly. This is because it is active during the day and has colourful patterns on its wings. It is considered to be one of the world's most beautiful insects.

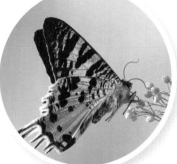

▲ *The flashy colours of the sunset moth are created by the curvature of the scales on their wings that reflect light in different angles*

◀ *The giant swallowtail butterfly feeding on a pink zinnia flower. They are some of the largest butterflies found in North America.*

▼ *Butterflies are attracted to specific types and colours of flowers*

Caterpillars Get Wings

A life cycle refers to the changes an organism goes through after it is born until it reaches adulthood. Some organisms, which include butterflies and moths, undergo a process called **metamorphosis**, which means that they go through so many drastic changes that they look completely different as adults than when they were newborns.

Egg

First, the male and female butterflies or moths have to find each other. They do so in varied ways. In cecropia moths, at mating time, females produce natural chemicals which are smelled by the males almost 2 kilometres away. The males use their feathery antennae to detect the smell. Once the male and female of the species mate, the female is ready to lay eggs.

The female butterfly or moth lays eggs on the underside of leaves or on stems. Usually, the eggs are laid on plants which are eaten by the new hatchlings, so that they do not have to go hunting for food. For example, the female brimstone butterfly lays eggs on buckthorn leaves. During the next stage, the caterpillars eat these leaves.

Eggs

Butterfly

Caterpillar

Pupa

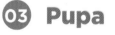
▲ *The life cycle of a butterfly*

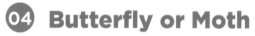 Butterfly or Moth

At last, the butterfly or moth is ready inside the pupa. The pupa breaks open, but the adult does not fly immediately. Its wings are still wet, wrinkled, and stuck to the body. The butterfly or moth waits for them to dry. To make them strong, the insect pumps a fluid called haemolymph into them. Once the wings are ready for flight, the butterfly or moth takes off.

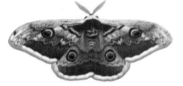
▲ *Moths are one of the largest pollinator groups besides bees and butterflies*

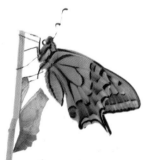
◀ *Butterfly emerging from pupa*

02 Caterpillar

The eggs hatch and the caterpillars emerge. As soon as they are born, they start eating a lot. During this phase, caterpillars moult several times. As a caterpillar grows its skin gets tighter and splits or cracks appear on the surface. After emerging from the egg, a caterpillar can grow up to 100 times its size. It is now ready for the next stage.

◀ *Caterpillars feed on plants such as cudweed, tulips, and black cherries*

03 Pupa

The caterpillar's next phase is not to be a moth or butterfly, but to change into an inactive, hard-cased pupa or chrysalis. It attaches itself to stems or twigs of plants. This stage lasts for days, even weeks depending upon the species. The hard case protects the budding butterfly inside from predators and extreme weather conditions. The caterpillar starts to develop legs, wings, and other organs that will make it a butterfly or moth.

This stage of the insect's life is quite crucial as it is essentially defenceless. Lots of caterpillars do not reach the next stage due to attacks from predators or other challenges such as harsh weather.

The Migratory Monarch

The regal-sounding monarch butterfly is an interesting insect. Not only does it migrate, but it also has an effective self-defence mechanism. The butterfly uses a chemical defence system. At the caterpillar stage, it eats milkweed plants, which contain toxic compounds called cardenolides. The toxins accumulate in its body, protecting it and subsequently the adult monarch from predators.

Appearance

The monarch is a stunning butterfly with orange wings marked with black veins and borders, and white spots. The wingspan of an adult monarch could be close to 12 centimetres. Between the male and female monarch butterflies, it is the females which have thicker veins on their wings. The colourful scheme helps ward off the predators.

Migration

Monarchs are not native to only Central, North, and South America, but are also found in Australia, India, parts of Europe, and some islands in the Pacific Ocean. The interesting thing about monarchs is that this migration is practiced only by the North American butterflies. Just before winter every year, hordes of these tiny butterflies get ready for migration. They leave their summer breeding grounds in the USA and Canada to travel more than 5,600 kilometres to reach southern California and central Mexico. It is said that millions of butterflies are a part of the migration. Most monarch butterflies return to the same woodland.

Unsolved Mystery

Monarchs survive for a few months. Towards the end of winter, the male and female monarchs in Mexico and California mate. The males die and females head northwards. On the way, they lay eggs on the milkweed trees and die. How the next generation knows where to go is still an enigma. The butterflies might have an internal compass that helps them reach the right place in the right season.

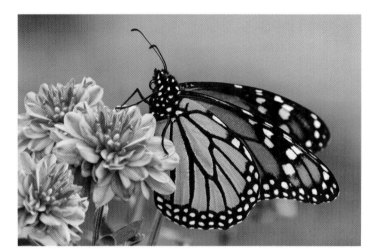

▲ A monarch butterfly resting on a flower

Under Threat

Since 1983, the International Union for Conservation of Nature (IUCN), a body that governs all animal and plant species around the world, has listed the monarch butterfly's migration as threatened. In Mexico, huge tracts of land, where these butterflies used to make their homes, were cleared of forests and replaced with plantations. Also, milkweed trees are reducing in number because of logging.

⭐ Incredible Individuals

A zoologist named Fred Urquhart (1911–2002) discovered where the monarch butterflies spent their winters in 1975. After his findings were published in the National Geographic, the government of Mexico demarcated certain areas in the country for the protection and conservation of these butterflies in 1979. However, Fred Urquhart started doing his research in 1937 and only completed it 38 years later. He worked with his wife, Norah Roden Urquhart, who tracked and tagged several butterflies for their research. He discovered several other facts about butterflies during his research. According to Urquhart, butterflies only take flight during the day, when there is sunlight. They can fly 130 kilometres in one day. Butterflies of all ages from different generations fly together during the migration period.

◀ Scientists are yet to unravel the mystery of the monarch migration

Jump and Chirp

Crickets and grasshoppers belong to the insect order Orthoptera. This is the same order that dragonflies, stoneflies, and cockroaches belong to. Most of these insects have the ability to camouflage so that they can blend into their surroundings.

The Hind Wonder

Have you ever tried to touch a grasshopper? If you have, you must have noticed the leaps it takes. Both crickets and grasshoppers have powerful hindlegs for leaping and jumping, usually to escape predators. As they leap, they spread their rear wings. The rear wings are larger, with a membrane, and are usually colourful. Both the insects have rigid forewings.

The Ear Tale

Grasshoppers and crickets have no ears. Instead they both have an organ—a stretched membrane of skin—called the tympanum. In case of crickets, it is located on the knee-like joints of their front legs, while in grasshoppers the membrane is located underneath the abdomen. The organ detects sound vibrations which are sent to the brain.

▼ *Grasshoppers existed long before dinosaurs*

Wings

Spiracles

Hindleg

Midleg

Sing a Song

The chirping of crickets and grasshoppers is a very familiar sound in summers, especially in cold regions. The noise created is not actual singing but is called **stridulating**. It is created by rubbing two body parts together. Crickets rub their front wings to create the sound, while grasshoppers rub their hindlegs against the front wings. Most often, the male insects sing. They do so to warn others off their territory or to attract mates.

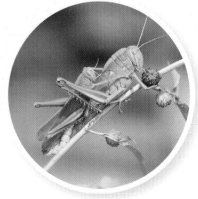

◀ *Most grasshoppers have a herbivorous diet*

▲ *Crickets have more protein than beef or salmon*

Katydids are a species of crickets. They make sounds just like crickets and grasshoppers. While the songs of most crickets get repetitive within a second, the song of katydids repeats in an alternating pattern. Different species also have their own songs. The US katydids are called virtuoso katydids for this reason. However, they perform at a high frequency, so people might not be able to hear their songs.

Amplified

The mole cricket is an interesting insect. Male mole crickets make special burrows during mating season. They dig two trumpet-shaped openings which act as megaphones. It is through these loudspeakers that they send across their mating calls. On a still night, these calls can be heard from almost 400 metres away.

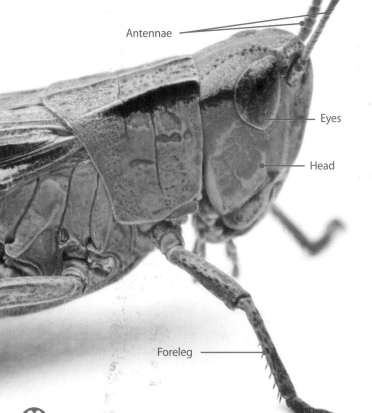

Antennae

Eyes

Head

Foreleg

On Hatching

The young **nymphs**, as they are called, of the grasshoppers and crickets look like smaller versions of the adults, except they lack wings. As the nymphs grow and shed their skin, the wings emerge slowly. With each successive moult the nymph resembles an adult more and more. This type of development, where there is no pupa stage, is called **incomplete metamorphosis**.

Crickets v/s Grasshoppers

Crickets and grasshoppers have certain dissimilarities which make it easy to tell them apart. Crickets have long antennae, while grasshoppers have short antennae. Crickets come out at dusk, but grasshoppers are active during the day. Crickets do not eat plants, but they can eat animals and each other. On the other hand, grasshoppers strictly rely on plants for food. An earwig is a small herbivorous, nocturnal insect belonging to the same family as the grasshoppers and crickets. It sprays a foul-smelling liquid to defend itself from predators, but it is harmless to us.

Mating

The perfect time to find mates is during summer, when the weather is warm. Grasshoppers and crickets turn to their musical abilities for this. Soon they get a mate to create the new generation. Most often, the adult insects in both types do not last the harsh winters, especially in colder climatic regions. It is only their eggs which survive the cold. However, in warmer regions the insects tend to survive longer.

Securing the Eggs

Female grasshoppers dig a hole in the ground, pushing the abdomen hard to release anywhere between 20–100 eggs. The eggs are covered with a white frothy liquid which solidifies to form a casing. It is this casing and the soil that protects the eggs throughout winter. Once the incubation period is over, tiny grasshoppers emerge from the eggs.

In case of crickets, the story is slightly different. Similar to the grasshoppers, female crickets dig holes in the soil, but here the female digs as many holes as the eggs she lays. The number of eggs is usually 100 and a single hole has a single egg. The eggs are protected by the soil in winters. After incubation, tiny crickets emerge from the eggs.

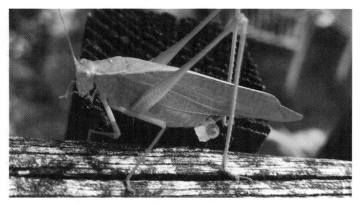

▲ *A grasshopper carefully laying eggs*

⊙ Incredible Individuals

Dr William H. Cade is a biologist who conducted research on field crickets and flies, as well as the evolution and reproduction habits of insects. He studied the acoustic signals of a cricket and the mating habits of cockroaches. In 1975, he made a discovery with his wife, Elsa Salazar Cade. They found that a female **parasitic** fly actually becomes attracted to the male cricket's song. They deposit larvae near these males. The larvae eat up the crickets within a week and enter the pupa stage. So, he discovered that these parasitic flies are the natural enemies of crickets.

The Mighty Dragonfly

Dragonflies are also called the devil's darning needle. They belong to the Odonata order of insects, which in Greek means the 'toothed one'. Yes, a dragonfly is known for its saw-like teeth. These insects have been around for almost 300 million years, but they have not changed much from their ancestors.

Tracing the Evolution

Insects first appeared about 380 million years ago at a time called the Devonian Period. They were small and wingless, without any developed legs. The next stage in evolution was the development of wings. The oldest fossil evidence dates back to the Carboniferous Period, which was 300 million years ago. It was then that the first dragonflies appeared. It is said that dragonflies grew to monstrous proportions, with a wingspan of almost two feet, as much as any modern bird.

▲ *Dragonflies reproduce by indirect insemination*

Modern Dragonflies

As they evolved, the dragonfly's wing size reduced to 2–15 centimetres, which is the same as the modern dragonfly. The wings are delicate, veined, and generally transparent with coloured markings. The dragonfly's body is long. The insect has two pairs of wings, one in the front and another in the back. Both the wing pairs are shaped differently. At rest, the wings do not fold close to the body but are spread out. Dragonflies have compound eyes that give them 360° vision to spot their prey as well as their predator.

Forewing

Hindwing

Thorax

Head

Foreleg

Hindleg

▲ *The dragonfly is small, but it has many complex parts*

Abdominal Segments

In Real Life

Do you know there roamed cockroaches three or four times as big as those present today? This happened during the Carboniferous Period. It is said that abundant swamps and forests created excess oxygen in the atmosphere. Oxygen, although an essential gas for survival, can lead to harmful effects if inhaled in excess. Small bugs could not have sustained the excess gas, so scientists theorise that they grew in size, in proportion to the amount of oxygen their bodies could take in for survival.

Flight of the Dragon

Dragonflies are experts in flying. They can move up, down, backwards, sideways, or hover like a helicopter. The interesting thing about this insect is that it usually catches its prey in mid-air. Small flying insects such as mosquitoes, bees, and butterflies are easy prey. Dragonflies have not changed their ancient flying technique. Their wings are controlled directly by their muscles. These sets of muscles contract and relax alternately, which pulls the wings up and down.

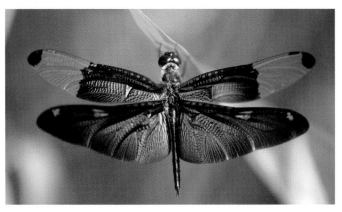

▲ *There are more than 5,000 known species of dragonflies*

Optimum Requirement

The muscles of dragonflies have to reach an optimum temperature before flight. Small dragonflies can take off with a body temperature of 12°C, but larger ones need a minimum temperature of 20°C. To reach these temperatures, the insects bask in the heat of the Sun or engage in rapid movement of their wings. If the insect overheats, it glides in the air to cool down.

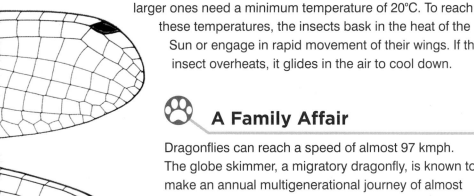

A Family Affair

Dragonflies can reach a speed of almost 97 kmph. The globe skimmer, a migratory dragonfly, is known to make an annual multigenerational journey of almost 18,000 kilometres. This means that generations of dragonflies take the journey together. On the way, the younger dragonflies breed, and the older generations die out.

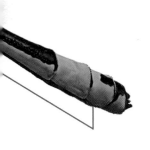

▶ *Despite having six legs, most dragonflies can barely walk*

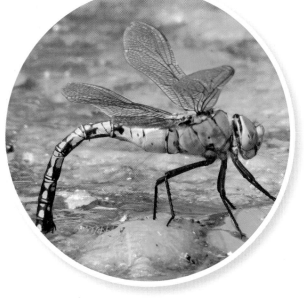

Isn't It Amazing!

The other name of the dragonflies, the devil's darning needle, comes from an old superstition. It was believed that these insects could sew up the mouth, eyes, and ears of sleeping children, especially, those who misbehaved. In reality, the dragonfly is harmless to human beings. In fact, human beings pose a bigger threat to their survival due to climate change.

▲ *Dragonflies can see even ultraviolet and polarized light*

Generation Next

Dragonflies live in areas with abundant water. First comes the egg stage. The female of the species lays the eggs in plant tissue, moist soil, and in water or on its surface. Depending on the incubation time of the dragonfly species (there exist close to 5,000 species of dragonflies in the world), the eggs hatch. The newly emerged nymph leads an aquatic existence. It is a voracious eater, preying on small fish, crustaceans, tadpoles, and worms.

The nymphs get oxygen through their gills located at the end of the digestive canal. Expanding and contracting their bodies, they force water through the gills. They swim in the same way, using the force of water. Depending on the species, the larvae moult a number of times. Eventually, they become beautiful adult dragonflies; these can lead an adult life spanning between 4 months to 10 years.

The Praying Mantis

The praying mantis, also known as *Mantis religiosa*, is a small but fierce hunter. It is known to take on animals much larger than its own size.

🐾 What's in a Name?

The praying mantis gets its name because of its long front legs. They are bent such that the mantis seems to be kneeling in prayer. This insect belongs to a bigger group of hunters called the mantids. Over 2,400 species species of mantids exist in the world.

🐾 Waiting for Prey

The praying mantis has a triangular head on which are perched two large compound eyes and three smaller simple ones between them. These eyes have blessed the insect with excellent vision. With its long neck, the insect can turn its head 180° to scan the surroundings.

While sitting on leaves, it is camouflaged properly because of its bright green colour. As it rests between the flowers and branches of a plant, the praying mantis waits for hours for its prey to appear. Once the prey comes closer, the praying mantis strikes with lightning speed and grabs the prey with its pincer-like spiny front legs. The rest of the four legs are used for walking.

🐾 Diet

The praying mantis is known to eat moths, crickets, and grasshoppers. Occasionally, it is known to eat very small birds such as hummingbirds and even reptiles. In Karnataka, India, a team of scientists discovered an adult praying mantis preying on small guppies, a type of fish swimming in a pond. To reach the fish, the insect used the floating leaves on the surface of the pond. Of course, the species was the giant rainforest mantis, which is said to be almost 7 centimetres in length.

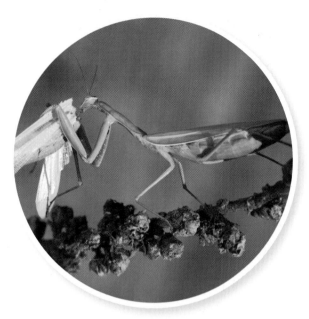

▲ *The praying mantis has a pair of antennae with which it navigates its surroundings*

🐾 Cannibalistic Females

Female praying mantises are interesting insects. To mate, the male has to hop on the female, but if it misses the jump, it becomes the female's next meal. Also, while mating, the female might devour the male's head. The body completes mating after which the rest of the dead male is eaten by the female.

Female praying mantises then lay 12–400 eggs in groups. These are surrounded by a liquid which hardens into a protective shell. The eggs spend the winter protected inside it, to emerge in spring. Infants need the entire summer to grow into adulthood. In case of infants too, many a time their first meal consists of their siblings. Otherwise their meal is fruit flies and very tiny insects.

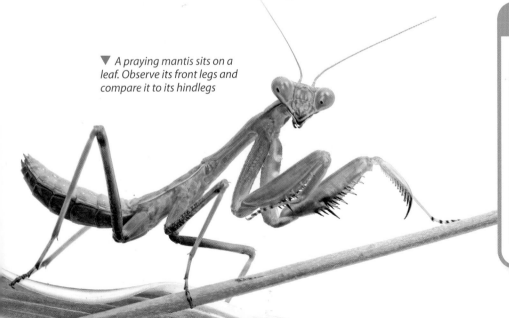

▼ *A praying mantis sits on a leaf. Observe its front legs and compare it to its hindlegs*

💡 Isn't It Amazing!

Praying mantises are associated with various religious and medicinal beliefs. In Greek they are known as 'mantes', which means prophet. In China, it is thought that these insects help in the cure of goitre, a **thyroid** problem. The Chinese believe that eating roasted eggshells of praying mantises prevents children from wetting their beds at night. These instances reflect how the insect features in various cultures.

The Hidden Sticks

Stick insects display some of the best camouflage in the world. They resemble twigs. Coincidentally, they also live amongst twigs, making them hard to spot. These insects come in varied sizes. Among the smallest is the 1.30-centimetre-long *Timema cristinae* of North America. Among the biggest is the 38.2-centimetre-long *Phryganistria chinensis* of Sichuan, China. With legs stretched, this insect measures a length of 64 centimetres, making it the longest insect in the world.

A Stick Story

Stick insects are usually green or brown in colour. Many have wings and few have spines. These spines are used in defence to prevent predator attacks. Some play dead to keep the attacker at bay, while few prefer to lose a leg in escape. Additionally, there is one species in North America which releases a foul-smelling liquid. These are nocturnal insects that spend their day motionless amongst plants.

Stick insects are commonly found in the tropics; however, few species also live in the temperate zones. They live in forests and grasslands, where they find ample vegetation to feed on.

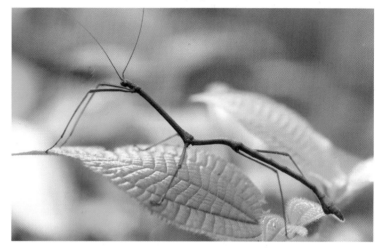

▲ *Stick insects can regenerate their limbs*

Howe a Stick Survived

Lord Howe Island stick insects are big (almost 15 centimetres long), flightless, nocturnal insects named after an island of the same name in the Pacific Ocean. They were first found on this island off the coast of Australia. They are usually blackish or dark brown in colour with a distinct abdomen and six long legs. Their size and appearance have given them nicknames such as land lobster and tree lobster. The young ones of these stick insects are called nymphs and they are green in colour.

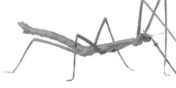

◀ *Ctenomorpha gargantua stick insects are bred in captivity to keep the species intact*

Mysterious Appearance

Lord Howe Island stick insects were once so abundant that fishermen used them as bait. A shipwreck and accidental introduction of rats on the island in 1918 wiped out the population of stick insects there. In the 1960s, these stick insects were thought to be extinct. But in 2001, as a miracle, they were found once again about 20 kilometres away from the island on a volcanic remnant called the Ball's Pyramid. How these flightless creatures reached there is a mystery.

These fall in the critically endangered list of the IUCN. Today it is said that only 30–40 survive in the wild. Fortunately, the Australian government is taking strict measures to safeguard and increase the remaining population.

In Real Life

Leaf insects belong to the same order as the stick insects, the order Phasmatodea. They are often called walking leaves because of their uncanny resemblance to a leaf. Many even have a vein structure similar to the leaves. The camouflage nature has created for them is simply stunning! These flat insects feed on plants and are found in the Indian Ocean, Southeast Asia, as well as Australia.

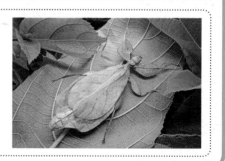

▶ *A leaf insect rocks back and forth to mimic a real leaf being blown by the wind*

A Historical Pest

Locusts and grasshoppers are cousins. A locust may look as harmless as its cousin on a bright summer morning, as it jumps plant to plant. But do you know a locust can be one of the most devastating insects on the planet?

Appearance

Similar to grasshoppers, locusts are green or tan in colour and have strong hindlegs which allow them to make strong jumps. They make a distinctive noise by rubbing their hindlegs together. They too have external mouth parts. They use their strong, toothed mandibles to cut and chew vegetation. The cut food is held and pushed up into the mouth with the help of pincer-like maxillae. A solitary locust leads a peaceful life. It is a shy creature.

Swarm Formation

Then there could come a phase, wherein the five-centimetre small locust undergoes a complete character change just like Dr Jekyll transforms into Mr Hyde. The locust can turn from good and peaceful to annoyed and vengeful. The most infamous of all species is the desert locust. They live in the desert areas between India and West Africa.

Especially after good rains, where there is a bounty of food, the desert locusts breed. As long as there is enough food for the entire population, the insects are happy. But the moment there is competition, the character of the insect changes. It enters into what is called the gregarious phase. Not just its behaviour, which becomes aggressive, its appearance too changes; it turns black and yellow. The insect is ready to swarm!

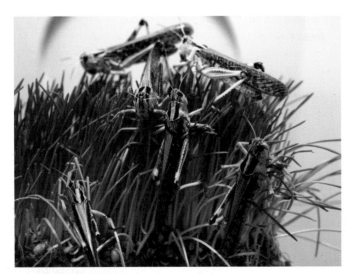
▲ Locusts have affected crops and farmlands since biblical times, attacking any grown green vegetation in their path

▲ Each locust can eat its weight in plants each day

A Long March

Desert-locust nymphs (young ones) will move about 300 metres daily to find food, but adult swarms can fly as much as 3,200 kilometres in one year, destroying vegetation along the way. Locusts usually migrate towards low pressure zones where rains are likely. In other words, they follow the rain patterns in the area they live in.

In Real Life

An adult locust can eat vegetation which equals its body weight. Take a guess at how much a small swarm of locusts can eat. It can eat enough food for 2,500 people. It can devastate entire fields within minutes. Swarms are capable of impacting the livelihoods of one-tenth of the people on the planet. In 2004, a swarm of locusts swept across Mauritania to Egypt and went further to Israel in the east and Portugal in the north. Of course, human beings are better equipped today to deal with the swarms than they were in the last century, thanks to improved monitoring and control techniques. But if the infestation goes undetected, it could be years before things are rectified at a cost of millions of dollars.

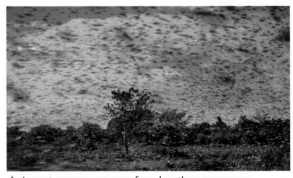
▲ Locust swarms can vary from less than one square kilometre to several hundred square kilometres

Unwelcome House Guests

External parasites are called ectoparasites. These ectoparasites mostly belong to the insect family. For a parasite living outside the host, the main problem is how to benefit from the host. It either has to stay attached or attach briefly to penetrate the host, at least while it is feeding. The hairy surfaces of mammals are accommodating of many an ectoparasite. A great example is the cat flea.

🐾 A Purry Foe

Fleas are small, wingless insects bearing many bristles and spines. Cat fleas are generally host specific, but are found on other animals such as dogs, leopards, civets, and foxes too, if the regular host is not available.

The cat flea has a compressed body that helps it move with ease along cats' fur. The mouthparts are specialised to suck blood while the hindlimbs are developed for jumping on and off the host. It has well-developed knee and hip joints. So it can jump vast distances, equivalent to a man jumping a multi-storey building. The hair on the body and legs stop the flea from falling off the cat's fur. The insect is known to survive on the cat's blood. It causes intense itching and inflammation on the cat's skin.

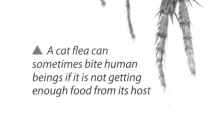

▲ *A cat flea can sometimes bite human beings if it is not getting enough food from its host*

🐾 A Wakeup Bite

Bedbugs are small insects with the appearance of an apple seed. They have flat, rust-coloured bodies. The adults are less than one centimetre long. These insects do not fly, but they can quickly crawl on surfaces. Their mouths are equipped to suck blood.

During the daytime, bedbugs are inactive, but at night they find human beings and suck on their blood. They feed for about 3–10 minutes. Their bodies swell and become bright red. Do you know these bugs can go without food for weeks at a stretch? At right temperatures, based on the availability of food, female bedbugs can lay close to 200–400 eggs.

Bedbugs do not kill human beings, but they lead to itching and red rashes on the skin. The infestation is commonly seen in the crevices of walls, furniture and of course, beds and mattresses, which is where they get their name from.

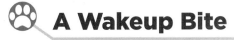

▲ *Bedbugs belong to order Heteroptera. These insects can live in almost any type of environment*

🐾 Sleeping Sickness

The tsetse fly, also known as the tik-tik fly, is a bloodsucking fly native to Africa. This yellowish brown or dark brown insect belongs to the housefly family. There are two distinguishing characteristics of the tsetse flies. One is the presence of a piercing, stiff mouthpart that can puncture skin. This is horizontal most times, but it becomes vertical when the insect wants to bite. The second is a bristle-like appendage on each antenna, which bears on its upper edge a row of long, branched hair.

Tsetse flies are known to suck the blood of human beings, as well as domestic and wild animals. In human beings, they cause a disease called sleeping sickness. It leads to muscle aches and fever. The infected person feels tired all the time. If the disease is not treated, it can enter the brain, leading to complications and difficulties in the treatment and cure.

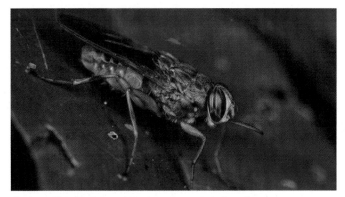

▲ *Tsetse flies are between 6–16 millimetres in length*

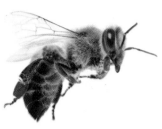

The Busy Bee

There exist close to 20,000 species of bees in the world. The Australian *Euryglossina* is just two millimetres long, while the Indonesian *Megachile* is almost four centimetres in length. The world of bees is diverse and colourful. The American sweat bee, attracted to perspiration, is green and blue. On the other hand, the valley carpenter bees have black-bodied females and yellow-bodied males.

Hive Building

Bees live in nests called hives. The central feature of the nest is the cell, a single structure in which the laid egg develops into the pupa. Only in social species, such as the honeybees, are these cells grouped together to form honeycombs, which are made of wax. In these cells, there are areas designated to bring up the young ones and store honey and pollen. Each cell is hexagonal.

Social Structure

In case of a solitary bee, nest-building is carried out by the mother with materials such as soil or wax, but in social bees, the hives are a very organised structure. Honeybee societies are perfectly organised with each 'caste', as it is called, performing its own task. Their tasks consist of three ranks—the smallest and most numerous are the worker bees. These are **sterile** females. Their main function is to build, maintain, and defend the nest.

The worker bees are all females, but do not lay eggs. Also, it is the worker bee which performs the famous dance of the bees, the 'waggle dance'. After a brief flight outside, when a worker bee returns to the hive, it dances to convey the direction in which food sources can be found in plenty.

Eggs are always laid by the queen bee. It is the largest bee in the entire hive and mother to all the workers. Finally, there is the drone bee, whose work is to mate with the queen bee to produce the next generation.

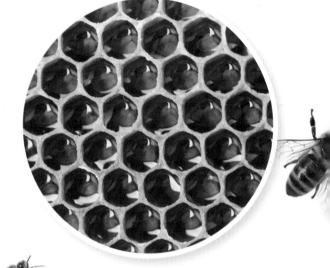

▲ *One bee colony can produce up to 150 kg of honey per year*

☀ Isn't It Amazing!

A honeybee can fly at a speed of 25 kmph and beat its wings almost 200 times per minute. Also, honeybees have close to 170 odour receptors, indicating that smell is important to them. Honeybees use this power to communicate and locate different flowers for food. They also help pollinate the flowers, helping in the process of reproduction by cross-pollination.

The Wax Factory

Wax is produced from the glands on the underside of the worker bees. The bee kneads the wax with its front legs and mouth parts, mixing it with its saliva to make it useable. What is interesting is the temperature of the nest, which is maintained at 45° C to keep the wax soft to work with. Along with the wax, the bees also produce a glue called propolis. It helps in plugging the gaps and cracks in the hive.

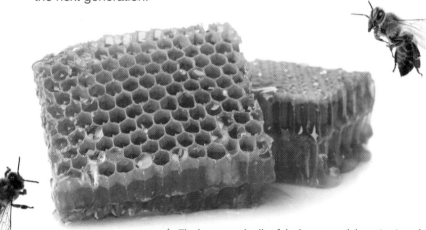

▲ *The hexagonal cells of the honeycomb have intrigued people since ancient times. It is an efficient shape that is also used by other insects such as the paper wasp*

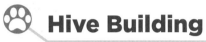

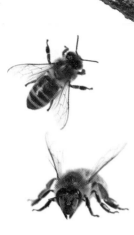

▶ *Most bees live a solitary existence. It is only a few such as the honeybees and bumblebees which lead a social life. In their colonies, they do not just live together but work together as well*

The Hive

There exist some honeybee hives that contain as many as 100,000 bees. The honeybee hives consist of a number of wax combs suspended from a structure like a tree or a wall. The cells at the borders of the hive contain nectar mixed with saliva. The workers fan this mixture to evaporate the water. The cells are then capped with wax and sealed. This mixture gradually turns into honey. Other cells are used to store pollen. Developing larvae in uncapped cells are looked after by the worker bees. They are fed honey and pollen. On becoming young adults, the bees emerge from the cells, which are cleaned by the worker bees for reuse. The queen lays eggs in the centre of the hive. Drones do not perform any household duties and are driven away in times of food scarcity.

Queen Bee

If the queen bee dies, the workers select a larva and feed it with what is called the 'royal jelly', a nutritious secretion. The larva then develops into the queen bee. She can live for up to 5 years and in summers can lay almost 2,500 eggs per day. She is vital to the functioning of the hive as it is she who directs the work and behaviour of the other bees, and maintains balance in the hive by allocating roles. She communicates all this through chemicals called pheromones, which dictate the behaviour of the bees.

Mistaken Identity

Wasps are close cousins of the bees. They look so similar that it is often a case of mistaken identity. But there are differences between the two insects. Honeybees have a light coat of hair which allows them to trap pollen. Wasps have little to no hair. While honeybees have rounded bodies, wasps have pointed bodies. Honeybees eat nectar, but wasps also eat larval secretions and other insects. Honeybees do not sting people unless they are threatened, but wasps often use their sting as the first defence. Another major difference is that the legs of a honeybee are hidden while flying, but wasps have their legs hanging out while flying.

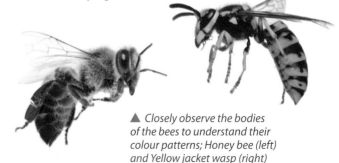

▲ *Closely observe the bodies of the bees to understand their colour patterns; Honey bee (left) and Yellow jacket wasp (right)*

The Useful Bee

The honeybee is one of the most useful insects out there. Apart from giving honey and beeswax to human beings, honeybees pollinate our crops. Pollination is the process of transfer of pollen from the anther of one flower to the stigma of another flower for fertilisation. On pollination, crops produce fruits and seeds.

Threatened Bees

A queen bee lives for about two to five years on an average, but recent trends show diminished longevity too. Also, colonies of honeybees are disappearing rapidly. The European honeybee is affected by 'colony collapse disorder', a condition characterised by the sudden death of colonies. The cause for the same remains a mystery.

Changes in the world of bees can drastically affect humans as well. One example of such change is the bee orchid pollinated by honeybees. Sadly, the plant is being forced to resort to self-pollination. The anther droops forward to contact the stigma of the same flower. This is common in the bee orchids in the far northern reaches of the planet; this has happened because the local population of honeybees there has almost become extinct.

Human Intervention

Honeybees are already reared commercially, but now their dwindling numbers demand our urgent attention. In places where the bee population has dropped down, farmers are resorting to hiring the services of beekeepers. How is this done?

A stack of hives is delivered to a farmer by a beekeeper. The keeper then releases the honeybees on the farm. The bees head towards the plants and begin the process of pollination.

In Real Life

The Asian giant hornets are huge wasps, as big as 5 centimetres long. Their sting is said to be very painful, and their swarms can decimate a beehive in a short time, killing all the bees inside. They then feast on the pupae and larvae. Their sting is fatal even to humans.

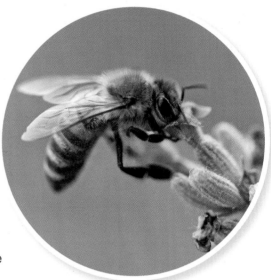

▲ One-third of the world's agricultural crop production depends on pollination

Beeswax

Beeswax is used to make candles, artificial fruits and flowers, furniture and floor wax, waxed paper, as well as cosmetics.

The Bumblebee

Bumblebees, also from the bee family, are fat and furry. They are found almost all over the world, except Antarctica. These bees are excellent pollinators. A single bee can visit close to 200 flowers in one trip to eat nectar, each time picking up and leaving behind a bit of the pollen. There are two types of bumblebees—those that build nests and those that are parasitic. There are several species of bumblebees that exist within these types. The average bumblebee is 1.5–2.5 cm in length.

◀ Bumblebees scent-mark the flowers that they have visited

Isn't it Amazing!

Plants do not release their entire nectar in one go. They release it in small amounts, encouraging bees to move from plant to plant, thereby aiding better pollination.

The Silk Road

There is a legend that says that around 3,000 years ago, the wife of Emperor Huangdi came across some threads. She decided to find the source of these threads, as she loved their texture. On searching for the source, she saw that worms living on white mulberry trees were producing the threads. She used the loom to produce lots of silk materials. However, this story might just be a myth. The origins of silk can certainly be traced back to China, but the exact details of this significant discovery are lost in the annals of history.

The Creator

Silk is produced by silkworms. But silkworms are not actually worms, as the name suggests. Instead, they are caterpillars of the silkworm moth. The silkworm caterpillar weaves threads around itself to form a cocoon as protection while it transforms to a moth during its pupa stage.

The silkworm moth has a wingspan that is about 5 centimetres long. It can have wings that look white or light brown in colour. The female silkworm moth is larger than the male. The sad part about these moths is that they live only for a few days. They do not eat in their lifetimes, as their mouth parts are either absent or reduced. They cannot fly either.

▲ *A silk moth lays up to 300 eggs at a time*

The Real Producer

Female silkworm moths produce about 300–500 eggs which hatch anytime between one to two weeks. The hatched larvae are less than one centimetre long. As soon as they are born, they start feeding on mulberry leaves, their preferred meal. They grow almost up to 7–8 centimetres long in 45 days. The cocoon they weave is of a continuous silk thread, either white or cream in colour, anywhere from 300–900 metres long.

▶ *Silkworms only eat mulberry leaves*

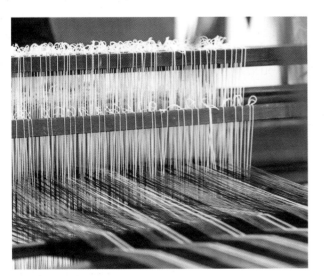

▲ *China is the the world's largest silk producer*

The Martyrs

Sericulture is the process of rearing silkworms and thereafter producing silk. So much domestication has taken place that there are almost no silkworm moths left in the wild anymore. Sadly, to create the shimmering, soft silk that humans love donning, caterpillars have to give up their lives. The first step in the production is to kill the pupae with steam or hot air. People for Ethical Treatment of Animals (PETA) and many other animal organisations have been protesting silk production for some time, but widespread use continues across the world. Silkworms have been **genetically modified** to create tougher and more elastic silk than that of the naturally domesticated variety. After silk threads are collected from the silkworm, they are spun and woven to create silk fabric.

The Builder Ants

Ants are insects that perhaps most human beings are familiar with. There are more than 12,000 species of these insects that exist today. They belong to the same insect order as wasps and bees—Hymenoptera.

The Slim One

Ants have a large head, elbowed antennae, and two sets of jaws; the front one to dig and carry food and the posterior one to chew the food. Ants are small, not more than 3 centimetres long. They come in varied colours, such as brown, red, yellow, and black.

Ants are known to 'hear' with their feet; the feet pick up the ground vibrations. Some such as driver ants have no eyes. In this case, they use their antennae to communicate. Also, they use chemical signals or pheromones to attract mates, warn others of danger, or convey the location of a food source. Ants eat nectar, seeds, fungus, and small insects.

Building a Society

Ant colonies come in varied sizes; they can range from a dozen individuals to a whopping one million of them living together. Similar to the bees, the ants show a structured society with each individual having a job based on its 'caste'.

The ant colony could have one or more queens. The queen lays eggs to create more and more members in the colony. The colony is teeming with worker ants, that are sterile females. There may be more than one type of worker, each performing a specific task. The young workers attend to the queen and look after the eggs and the smallest larvae. The middle-aged workers tend to the larger larvae and pupae, while the oldest of the workers guard the nest and hunt for food. The colony also has soldier ants with large heads and strong jaws for defending the colony.

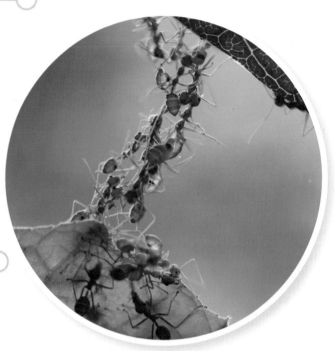

▲ *Armies of ants are known to attack and prey on reptiles, small birds, and even small mammals*

▶ *Ants can be found on every single continent except Antarctica*

Starting a Colony

A colony of ants has males too. At a certain time of the year, male ants and new queens are produced. These are winged adults, unlike the wingless workers. When the environmental conditions are right, the males and the queen leave the nest in a swarm. All ant nests in the area will swarm at the same time to ensure that ants from different parents mate. On mating, the male ants die, while the queens find a suitable nest; once inside, she pulls off her wings, lays eggs, and tends to the brood. When the workers emerge, the nest building begins.

Builders

Ants build nests in varied ways. Some use their jaws to shovel soil around the nest to form volcano-like craters. Some build mounds which they cover with loose vegetation; these mounds help regulate the temperature within the nests. An interesting feature of ants is that the nests are not temperature controlled; the insects move the eggs, larvae, and even themselves to where the temperature is suitable within the nest.

Not all ant nests are underground. In tropical regions, some ants are seen building their nests on trees. These nests are built with paper-like substances made with soil or wood and glued together with sugar solutions produced by ants.

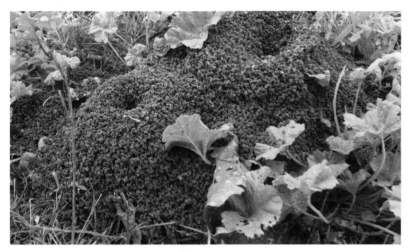

▲ The largest ant nest ever found is over 3,700 miles wide

Traits and Behaviours

Harvester ants often live in areas which are drought prone. To ensure supply of food in times of scarcity, they build vast underground storage areas where seeds are dried and kept. Tailor ants (also known as weaver ants) live on trees and as the name suggests they sew their nests. Large workers fold a leaf with their jaws and feet.

The European garden ant nests in rotting tree logs, under stones, or in loose earth. The main nest is underground and is made up of a series of chambers. When the Sun warms one part of the nest, the eggs and larvae are carried to that part. In winter, the entire colony transfers itself to the interior of the nest.

The Leafcutter ants, on the other hand, feed on fungi, which they culture inside their chambers. How do they do it? The ants cut pieces of leaves and carry them inside the nest. The leaves are chewed upon to help fungus grow on them. This is then eaten by the Leafcutter ants.

In Real Life

Do not disturb the colony of North America's red imported fire ants. They sting so hard that one needs to visit a doctor to get relief. Also, the ants cause a lot of damage to crops. This is not an insect one feels happy to have around!

Usefulness

Ants play an important role in recycling nutrients in an ecosystem. They do so by feeding on and breaking down small animals, other invertebrates, and plants. In the process of building homes, they 'till' the soil, which means they bring up the deeper layers of soil to the surface. These layers, with nutrients intact, are used by plants for growth.

Ants feed on the eggs of other insects but also, they are prey for lizards and birds. The tunnels they build aerate the surrounding soil. In fact, all of this digging helps them store the seeds that fall off of fruits and other plants. But ants can also cause damage. If their population is left unchecked, they can also destroy plants.

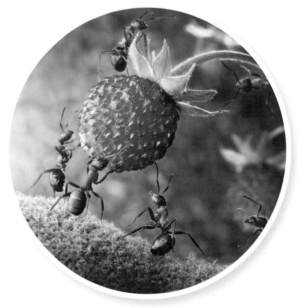

▲ Ants have superhuman strength! They can carry 10–50 times their body weight!

◄ Ants hold the record for the fastest movement in the animal kingdom

The Active Termites

Termites, another set of social insects, are found mainly in the warmer parts of the world. They are **xylophages**, which basically means that they are wood-eaters. Termites are known to damage thousands of trees every year. But they are also quite useful. Termites play an important role in decomposing plants and breaking down nutrients. They can do so because they have bacteria in their stomach which allow them to digest wood. These soft-bodied insects, unlike ants, do not have a waist. Their antennae are a series of segments. Many species of this small, pale insect are completely blind. There are around 2,000 species of termites in existence in this world.

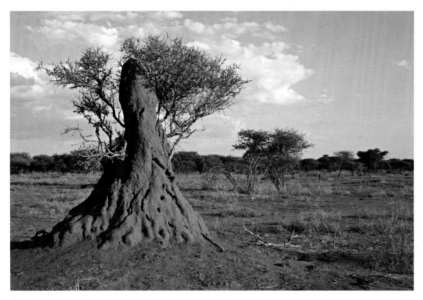

▲ Termite mounds can be up to 30 ft high!

Building Material

The main building materials in several species of termites that build big homes are soil and saliva. The second type of building material is carton, made up of a mixture of saliva and faecal remains and is used to build walls within the nest.

Mounds of termites are a common site in the African savannah. One species found there is the *Macrotermes natalensis*. These termites are capable of building homes with arches, an incredible feat of architecture for such a small insect. These arches provide a good air-conditioning system inside the nest. This type of nest has close to 2 million termites at one time and could take years to be built.

Termite nests need to accommodate a large number of insects living together, and it is for this reason that their mounds can reach heights of 17 feet and higher. The average termite mound can have around 15 kilograms of termites. In a typical year, these insects move almost 250 kilograms of soil and several tons of water.

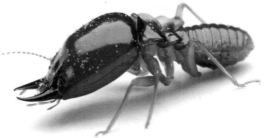

▶ Termites have been nicknamed 'silent destructors' by human beings because they can eat through paper and wood in a person's house without detection

A Model Home

Termite nests vary in size and shape. Some rise like castles above the ground, complete with chimney-like turrets, while others hang from trees. *Cubitermes* have mushroom-shaped homes, while another species, the *Thoracotermes* have straight pillar-like homes.

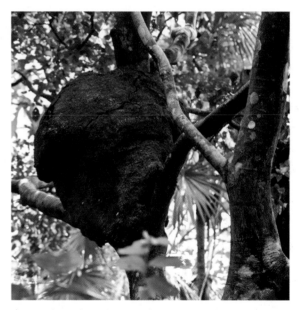

▲ An arboreal termite nest. These nests are brown and have little bumps on the outside

Isn't It Amazing!

Neocapritermes taracua are termites found in South America. They have an interesting defence mechanism. The aged workers of the colony grow sacs which are filled with a toxic, blue liquid. When they feel that the colony is threatened or a predator approaches, these sacs explode. They sacrifice their lives for the nest.

The Home Makers

In contrast to bees and ants, termite colonies contain an equal number of males and females, most of which are sterile. These are further divided into two categories; the regular workers and the soldiers. The soldiers do not look for food. They are fed **regurgitated** food; instead their duty is to guard the nest.

The workers are divided into two parts. The bigger ones are sent to forage for food, while the smaller ones build and repair the nest, look after the young ones, other members, as well as the royal couple.

There is usually a single royal couple in the colony. The king or the male is not as large as the queen or the female. The queen's abdomen increases dramatically in size during the egg-laying stage. The queen can lay as many as 30,000 eggs per day. The young ones born are a part of the same colony.

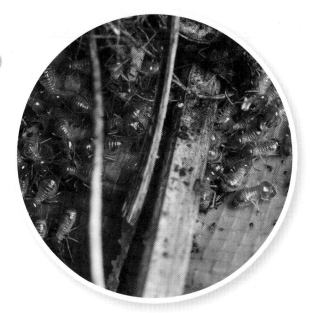

▲ Termite and ant colonies sometimes go to war over territory and access to food

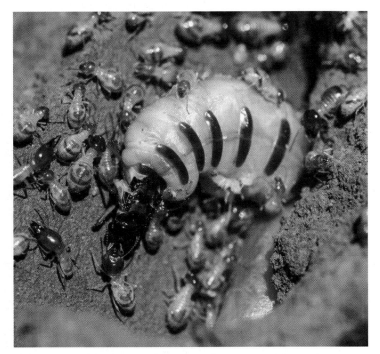

▲ Termite queens have the longest lifespan of any insect in the world—25–50 years!

⊙ Incredible Individuals

We know a lot about termites and their homes because of scientists. In fact, a group of scientists once prepared 500 different termite nests. These were simulated nests. They compared them to real termite nests and found that termites design everything of value within close distances. This is to ensure fast transportation. A scientist named J. Scott Turner experimented with termite nests or termite mounds by filling them with propane, stuffing them with plaster and scanning them with lasers. He even fed the termites microscopic beads and gave them fluorescent green water. He did all this to figure out how termites built their massive nests.

New Homes

Every termite colony has alates—temporarily winged males and females. A new termite colony is set up by the alates. The male is attracted to the female by an odour produced by the female; she has a gland meant for this on the underside of her belly. When the weather conditions are conducive, the alates swarm. Similar to ants, colonies of the same termite species in the area swarm at the same time, allowing breeding between individuals born to different parents. The temporary wings help young adults take flight; they then find their mates. Once on the ground, they shed their wings, build a small nest and seal themselves inside to mate and start a new colony.

Termites use different materials to build their homes. They mark all their construction materials with chemicals that they themselves produce. These chemicals dissolve over time. New chambers can emerge from the tunnels that they build in their homes. As the chemicals dissolve, termites can even make out if the chambers are old or new.

The Fungal Story

Macrotermes natalensis is a fungus-growing termite species commonly found in South Africa. These termites prefer dead plant material which has been made soft by fungus. In the dry season, the food supply diminishes as fungus needs humid conditions to thrive. To avoid this situation, the termites create fungus chambers with the help of carton. The fungus grows well in the humid atmosphere of the nest, giving enough food to the insects. Few of the termites from this species dig deeper to find water, so that it provides humid conditions for the fungus to thrive.

The Dangerous Mosquito

If you have ever sat outside on a summer evening, especially in the tropics, you will be familiar with this little pest. They create small red spots where they bite, and you are left scratching the spot. They don't just attack in the evenings, mosquitoes can be a menace at any time of the day. They do not just bite, but can also cause death, though not directly. Just three species of this insect are enough to wreak havoc on humans.

Bite

The body of a mosquito, when feeding, swells to such an extent that its skin stretches and becomes transparent enough for us to see the human blood inside. The mosquito's mouthparts are adapted for piercing the human skin. They consist of four **stylets** to pierce the skin. While biting, they stab two tubes into the victim. One is to pump in anti-coagulants which prevent the victim's blood from clotting and another is from which the blood is sucked.

Mosquitoes use a few signals to spot their victims, such as exhaled carbon dioxide, body odours, and even movement. Both male and female mosquitoes eat nectar and other sugars from plants. It is only the females which bite, since they use it as a source of protein to lay eggs.

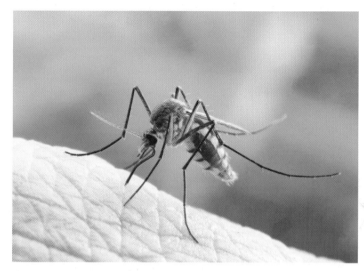

▲ Mosquito bites can cause many diseases, such as malaria, dengue, etc.

The Deadly Threesome

Mosquito-borne diseases are so prevalent that they are amongst the first priority of the World Health Organisation (WHO) as well as governments of countries affected. The deadliest are the following three types—the Anopheles, which is known to cause malaria as well as transmit filariasis and encephalitis; the Aedes, which spreads dengue, yellow fever, and encephalitis; and lastly the Culex, which causes filariasis, encephalitis as well as West Nile virus.

Vector

Did you know that the mosquito does not inherently have such disease-causing abilities? It is merely the vector, in other words carrier, of microorganisms which cause these diseases. In case of malaria, the plasmodium parasite attaches itself to the gut of the female mosquito. The moment the mosquito stings the victim for blood, it releases itself into the blood of the victim. Similarly, in dengue and yellow fever, the mosquito is the carrier of viruses that cause the diseases.

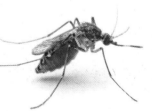

▲ Mosquitoes have a nerve that indicates when the stomach is filled; otherwise it would not stop drinking and burst from the pressure

Prevention

It is possible to control the spread of such diseases by controlling the vector. One important method is to destroy the mosquito in its larval stage itself. Mosquitoes need water to breed; especially if the water is stagnant, the larvae breed undisturbed. Careful monitoring of such sites has helped control the menace to a great extent in many African and Southeast Asian countries. Another method is to kill adult mosquitoes using insecticides.

⊛ Incredible Individuals

Charles Louis Alphonse Laveran (1845–1922) was a French doctor who found out the causal agent of malaria. While serving in Algeria, he was troubled by the outbreak of malaria in the army. While others blamed bad air ('*mala aria*' in Italian), he followed Louis Pasteur's line of thought which dictated that most infectious diseases are a result of germs. By 1880, he had enough evidence to prove that malaria was caused by mosquitoes that he won the Nobel Prize in Physiology or Medicine in 1907.

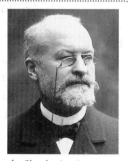

▲ *Charles Louis Alphonse Laveran*

The Irksome Housefly

Houseflies are a regular feature of our world. There are over 110,000 species of flies, out of which houseflies are just one. They live in almost all environments, except Antarctica.

Distribution

Houseflies are attracted to a range of things including water, exposed food particles, garbage as well as carrion. The latter two, garbage, and carrion, are certainly full of many infectious microorganisms; when the fly sits on them, its feet pick them up. Now, if the fly's next stop is exposed food, it transfers the microorganisms to the food. Once human beings consume this food, it leads to a variety of diseases such as cholera, diarrhoea, and typhoid.

▲ Houseflies rely on their sense of smell when they search for food

A Fly's Body

Houseflies are dull grey in colour with yellowish areas on the abdomen and grey stripes on the thorax. They are less than 1 centimetre long. What is interesting is that the housefly uses only one pair of wings in flight. This is because the second pair is reduced to knob-like structures called halters. It is these that help the housefly maintain balance while flying. Houseflies have huge compound eyes, which give them better vision.

▲ Houseflies' amazing eyes allow them to see behind them

Upside Down

At the end of the housefly's feet there are sharp claws and lots of sticky hair. This is because of the secretions produced by small glandular pads present between each claw on the feet. The claws and feet help the housefly hold onto surfaces when it is upside down. Also, being light in weight helps their bodies to hold on without falling.

Sponge-like Mouths

The short feelers of houseflies act like their nose. Once they pick up the smell of an object, they fly towards it. They use their feet hair to find out how something tastes. If they like it, their sponge-like mouthparts lap it up. Due to the soft mouthparts, a housefly cannot bite.

The Egg Story

A female housefly deposits close to 100 eggs at one time. In her lifespan she can produce up to 1,000 eggs. The eggs hatch anytime in the span of 24 hours. The housefly eggs undergo complete metamorphosis, which means they go from being larva to pupa to an adult. A housefly can live for a month or two.

Isn't It Amazing!

The fruit fly (*Drosophila melanogaster*) is the most-studied multicellular creature in the world. Thomas Hunt Morgan (1866 –1945) chose it as a 'model organism' for research in genetics—the study of genes. Fruit flies have a lifecycle of 10 days, and can be grown in glass bottles. By studying thousands of mutant flies, we have learnt a lot about how our genes guide our development.

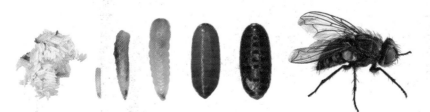

▲ Houseflies mostly breed on trash cans, animal dung, human excrement, decaying vegetable, and animal materials

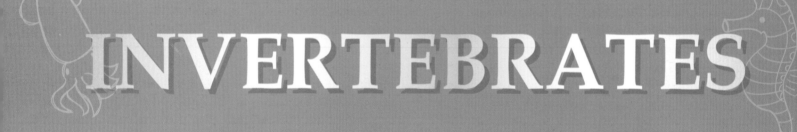

INVERTEBRATES

SPINELESS **WONDERS**

The term 'invertebrate' refers to living organisms without any vertebrae or backbone. These are amongst the oldest forms of living organisms, having evolved millions of years before the first vertebrates—the fish. But this life form still survives!

In fact, invertebrates not only survive, they thrive. Invertebrates account for almost 97 per cent of animals on Earth. Diversity, varied reproductive methods, and adaptability have made them some of the most resilient creatures on this planet. They are found in nearly every habitat, all in between hot and cold, from high to low. Turn the page to read about the amazing lives of invertebrates!

▼ *The sea sponge is a perfect example of an invertebrate*

Evolution of Invertebrates

The story of Earth began 4.5 billion years ago. That is a time beyond imagination. The planet was not as we see it today. It was uninhabitable due to high temperatures, volcanic eruptions, and collisions with other objects from the newly formed solar system. As time passed by, the planet stabilised. In the course of events, it gave rise to life.

First Life Forms

The first definite fossil evidence of life dates back to 3.5 billion years ago. Life originated in an atmosphere rich in methane and carbon dioxide, but very little oxygen. The first forms were **single-celled bacteria**. Fast forward to 2.3 billion years ago and a new type of bacteria evolved, called the cyanobacteria. It was unique as it produced oxygen through a process known

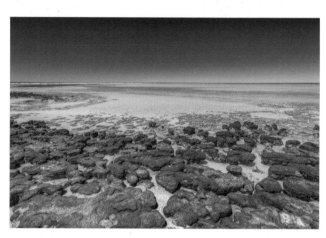

▶ The fossils of photosynthetic bacteria found in ancient rocks are called Stromatolites

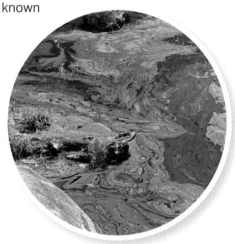

▲ The chlorophyll-rich cyanobacteria coat the river with green colour. These are tough creatures, still surviving on Earth in large numbers

Snowball Earth

Photosynthesising bacteria or cyanobacteria flourished and created more and more oxygen. This changed the atmosphere, making it rich in oxygen; while most of the earlier bacteria that depended on methane died out. Then, around 715–660 million years ago, Earth cooled down to such an extent that the temperatures at the equator dropped down to -20° C. This event is called 'Snowball Earth' and is thought to have been triggered by the rapid weathering of continents, which sucked out atmospheric carbon dioxide. Life could not sustain on this snowball. It was wiped out, except for the areas near deep-sea volcanic vents.

Cambrian Explosion

About 560 million years ago, the conditions changed and the environment became more habitable—a warm Earth, rising sea levels and of course, generous oxygen levels (a result of the cyanobacteria), lead to the creation of many new life forms. This time period is called the Cambrian Explosion. It was here that the first invertebrates appeared on Earth.

Trilobites

Trilobites are the icons of the Cambrian seas. As the name suggests, trilobites had three segments. They had tough, plated bodies to protect themselves from predators in the seas, and could grow as much as two feet in length. More than 17,000 species survived for millions of years, only to be wiped out at the end of the Permian Period, 251 million years ago. A few of these species were predators and some were scavengers. Many of them ate plankton. All trilobites had antennae and legs.

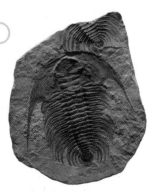

▲ Trilobites are among the most prolific fossils found in the seas

Isn't It Amazing!

Opabinia, belonging to an extinct group of animals called *Opabinia regalis*, swam the Cambrian seas. This creature had five eyes and caught its prey with a flexible claw-like arm that jutted out of its head. It stayed close to the seafloor, hunting ancient sponges for food.

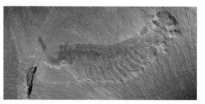

▲ A fossil specimen of the ancient invertebrate Opabinia regalis

🐾 Ancient Creatures

Following the Cambrian explosion, the seas were flooded with a variety of marine invertebrates along with trilobites. These were the graptolites, brachiopods, echinoderms, molluscs, corals and cephalopods. Many of these invertebrates were strange creatures. For example, the orthocone, a tailless, finless animal, was shaped like a long ice cream cone with tentacles. This 11-metre-long animal cut through waters hunting for prey such as the early species of fish and sea scorpions.

▲ A creature called Cameroceras had a unique shape which helped it jet-propel through the waters

🐾 Graptolites

Graptolites lived in colonies. They had tentacles and a **chitinous** outer covering. Most of these animals have been preserved as carbon impressions on shale, a type of a sedimentary rock.

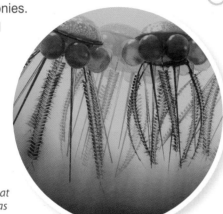

▶ A colony of graptolites that looked like floating umbrellas in the ancient sea

🐾 The Pterygotus

Pterygotus, a distant relative of the modern horseshoe crab, was a giant sea scorpion with some species measuring the length of almost eight feet. They were fearsome predators, holding onto their prey, such as early vertebrates as well as other sea dwellers, with their huge pincers. Apart from the pterygotus, almost 200 species of these extinct invertebrates have been identified. The fossils of these animals have been found in brackish and freshwater.

▲ An artist's rendition of the pterygotus

🐾 Devonian Period

Plants evolved much earlier than first thought by scientists. By the Devonian Period, which was about 416 million years ago, terrestrial vegetation started to spread. These plants did not have roots and shoots. They did not grow more than a few centimetres tall. Dwelling amongst these early plants were mainly arthropods in the form of insects, mites, and **myriapods**. So, the first insects had already evolved a few million years before the Devonian Period began. The early insects were small, wingless, and had simple antennae.

The shallow waters of the Devonian Period saw the development of large coral reefs. The seas continued to be populated by early invertebrates. However, by the end of the Devonian Period, most trilobite species had disappeared.

🐾 Passage of Time

Many large invertebrates like the *Arthropleura* grew to their size because there was more oxygen in the environment and fewer vertebrate predators on land. Eventually, these giant invertebrates reduced in size and modern arthropods came into being. It is their adaptability to the changing environment that has made invertebrates a lasting group of animals on this planet. These wonderful creatures were there before us and, according to scientists, will remain even after human beings have disappeared from Earth.

🐾 Carboniferous Period

About 360 million years ago during the Carboniferous Period, because of the growth of vast swamp forests, there was a tremendous rise in the levels of oxygen in the atmosphere. This rich oxygen-fed air allowed the arthropods to grow to humungous sizes. Arthropleura, for example, grew to almost 2 metres in length and close to 46 centimetres in width. One of its species is considered to be the largest terrestrial invertebrate ever.

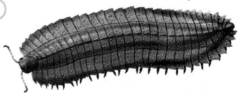

▲ The body of the Arthropleura had 30 segments like many modern millipedes

Tough Invertebrates

According to theories, invertebrates should have been the weakest of all organisms living on Earth. They lack backbones, only a few amongst them have a proper digestive system and many, such as sponges, do not even have brains and the associated intelligence. But in reality, invertebrates are among the toughest organisms on the planet. Read on to find out why.

Unchanged Invertebrates

In the course of evolution, some species of invertebrates have remained unchanged for millions of years and are surviving happily. These are the dragonflies and horseshoe crabs. However, fruit flies are still undergoing evolution. These flies are known to make simple changes in their genetic make-up over time. These changes help them survive changing environments.

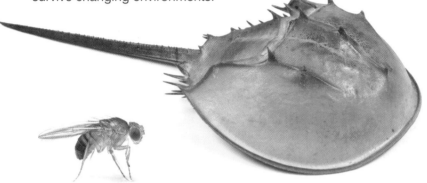

▲ Fruit flies have adapted to survive over time

▲ The horseshoe crab has resisted evolution. They are seen on seashores. If the coming waves flip them over, they use their long tails to flip back

Evolution of Resistance

The evolution of resistant, encapsulated dormant forms of invertebrates has enabled many among their species to survive in extreme conditions. For example, the eggs of freshwater fairy shrimp can remain dormant for months in dried mud, hatching only when the mud is submerged in the water again. These eggs are so resistant that even when exposed to temperatures as high as 99°C and as low as -190° C in laboratories, they have remained completely viable.

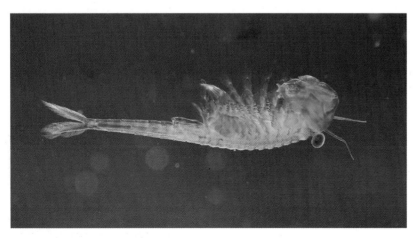

▲ Fairy shrimp have egg sacs near their tails

Breathing Methods

Earthworms need oxygen for survival, akin to human beings, but they have no lungs to gulp in air like human beings. That is why they breathe through their moist skin. But how do they maintain this moist skin? Not only do they live in damp soil, but their skin is also covered with a thin cuticle and slimy mucus.

Some spiders and scorpions have an interesting apparatus through which they breathe. They are called book lungs, which are a series of membranes that resemble the pages of a book. In between these membranes are air sacs which allow the air to circulate. Aiding the breathing process is the haemolymph, which is similar to the blood of human beings. For many insects, the trachea is the most important respiratory organ. This is usually made up of branching tubes. The trachea sends oxygen to all the tissues in the insect's body and takes away the carbon dioxide. The trachea is modified in insects that have to spend some time underwater. This allows them to exchange gases while they are underwater. These insects are called bubble breathers and the water beetle is the best example.

💡 Isn't It Amazing!

Haemolymph, a fluid equivalent to blood in most invertebrates consists of necessary nutrients which help the organism survive, but insects lack red blood cells as well as haemoglobin, giving haemolymph an almost colourless appearance.

Comb Jelly

The freely swimming comb jelly maintains its spherical shape through the presence of water in the internal canals. These canals support eight rows of comb plates, with which the comb jelly swims. Each comb plate is covered with hair-like cilia which propel the organism forward. The organism swims mouth-first.

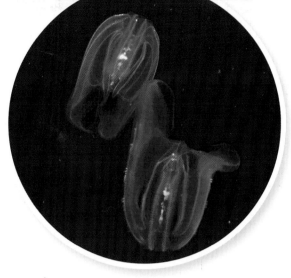

▶ Comb jellies are 95 per cent water

Structure

The stony coral polyp obtains support from a mineralised theca or a cup which is secreted by the animal. This helps anchor it to the basal structure of the coral colony as well as to its neighbours.

The closely related sea anemone does not use a rigid structure like the stone coral. Instead, it supports itself by using the water circulating around its central cavity. The water is drawn in through grooves on the sides of the cavity and expelled up the centre. It helps the organism maintain shape and internal pressure.

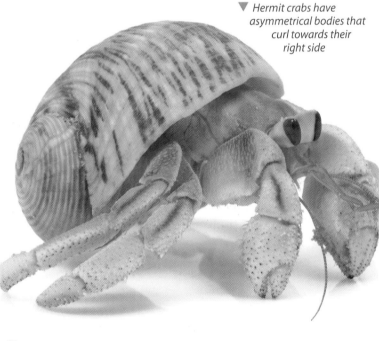

▼ Hermit crabs have asymmetrical bodies that curl towards their right side

Protective Armour

Invertebrates that are arthropods or joint-legged animals, such as scorpions, crabs, lobsters, and spiders have hard, chitinous, water-resistant exoskeletons which protect them from dehydration and various environmental changes such as extreme heat or heavy rains, as well as predators. This exoskeleton is moulted regularly by the invertebrate; it is while the exoskeleton is growing back that the invertebrate, with its exposed softness, is most vulnerable.

Molluscs such as snails have developed shells for protection, while hermit crabs live in discarded sea shells that wash up the shore, moving to a bigger one as they grow. But what is interesting is that this crab always finds an empty shell; it never kills or throws out the occupants of the shell.

Symmetry

Symmetry is the proportionality or evenness that is displayed on animal bodies. Most invertebrates are divided into three types of symmetries, namely bilateral symmetry, radial symmetry, and asymmetry. In bilateral symmetry, the body is divided into two equal parts by an imaginary line. Beetles, crabs, and lobsters have bilateral symmetry. In the case of radial symmetry, the body is oriented in a way that an imaginary line radiates through its centre, like in animals such as jellyfish and starfish. Asymmetrical organisms, such as sponges, are those with no symmetry; the body parts in such organisms do not correspond with each other to create a defined shape.

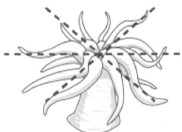

▲ A coral polyp has radial symmetry

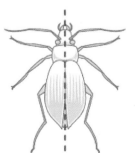

▲ A beetle has bilateral symmetry

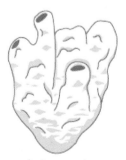

▲ A sponge has no symmetry

The Invertebrate Family

Jean-Baptiste Lamarck (1744–1829) was a French biologist who coined the term 'invertebrates'. Under this category, he put together all animals that lack the spinal cord. Invertebrates as a group include not just simple life forms such as sponges, but also the complex arthropods. There are more than 30 phyla or groups into which invertebrates are categorised. The major phyla are listed below. Insects, arachnids, molluscs, crustaceans, and their species belong to the group of invertebrates. They include animals that live on land and water.

01 Phylum: **Porifera**

Characteristics: Primitive; asymmetrical; filter out water for food particles; have no tissues but have specialised cells

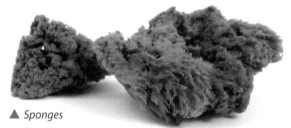

▲ Sponges

02 Phylum: **Cnidaria**

Characteristics: Aquatic; free-swimming life forms with radial symmetry; presence of tissues; incomplete digestive system

▶ Jellyfish

▼ Corals

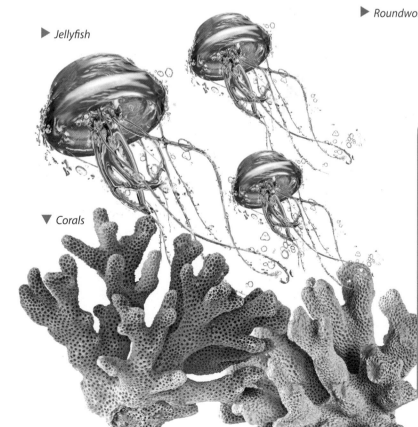

03 Phylum: **Platyhelminthes**

Characteristics: Aquatic and terrestrial habitats; soft-bodied; bilateral symmetry; incomplete digestive system; have a single opening to take in food and expel waste; **cephalisation**

▶ Fluke

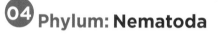

▲ Flatworm

04 Phylum: **Nematoda**

Characteristics: Aquatic and terrestrial habitats; bilateral symmetry; complete digestive system; have an excretory tube to remove waste

▶ Roundworms

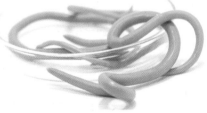

👆 In Real Life

Do you know what a body cavity is? It is a fluid-filled space not referring to blood or lymph vessels. Human beings have several body cavities. Flatworms have a gut, but no other body cavities. There are several smaller invertebrates that do not have any body cavity. As a result, the gut in bigger flatworms sends food to all body parts and makes their body shape flat. They also do not have an anus, which is used to remove waste. Flatworms can be free-living or parasitic. They are the largest phylum of the acoelomates, having nearly 25,000 species within the phylum.

05 Phylum: **Molluscs**

Characteristics: Aquatic and terrestrial habitats; have an organ system; body has a head, a foot and a **visceral** mass; have a true **coelom** and soft bodies which are at times covered with a hard exoskeleton; few have a primitive brain

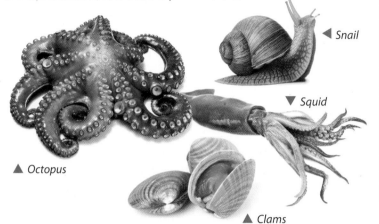

▲ Octopus

◀ Snail

▼ Squid

▲ Clams

06 Phylum: **Annelida**

Characteristics: Aquatic and terrestrial habitats; segmented bodies; coelomates; have a primitive brain

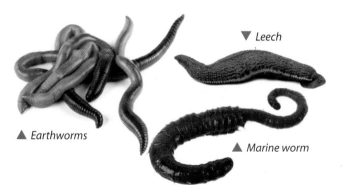

▼ Leech

▲ Earthworms

◀ Marine worm

07 Phylum: **Echinodermata**

Characteristics: Have an organ system with a complete digestive system and brain; presence of a spiny external covering as well as an internal skeleton; most have a **pentamerous** radial symmetry, i.e., they can be divided into 5 equal parts

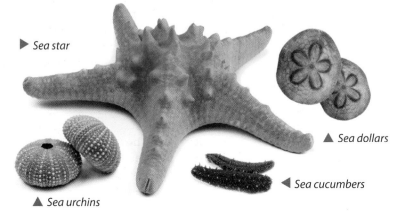

▶ Sea star

▲ Sea dollars

◀ Sea cucumbers

▲ Sea urchins

⊛ Incredible Individuals

While Charles Darwin (1809–1882) is credited with the theory of evolution, the idea behind this theory developed well before him in the 1700s. Jean-Baptiste Lamarck also put forth a theory of evolution of his own. He was a botanist who later became an expert on invertebrates and other boneless animals. In his research, he also realised that several animals shared similarities. He confirmed this observation by studying fossil records. He realised that as the environment changed, animals adapted to survive. He used the giraffe as an example of the same. He proposed that giraffes might have developed longer necks and front limbs as a result of a sustained habit of stretching to reach higher leaves on trees.

08 Phylum: **Arthropoda**

Characteristics: Bilateral symmetry; body divided into head, abdomen, and **thorax**; chitinous exoskeleton; joint appendages; presence of a proper brain compared to earlier phyla

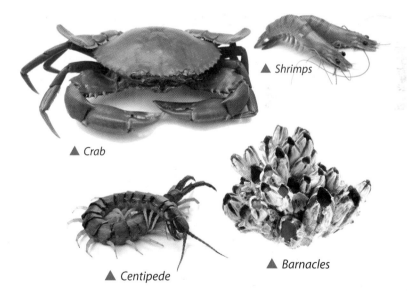

▲ Shrimps

▲ Crab

▲ Centipede

▲ Barnacles

🐾 **Secret for Success**

Invertebrates might have everything else going against them, but the big secret behind their successful life and evolution is their rate of reproduction. Some invertebrates, such as sponges can produce eggs and sperm themselves. Some other invertebrates do not need their eggs to undergo fertilisation; these include ants and bees. Invertebrates, especially insects, adapt easily.

Chemical Warfare

Invertebrates have one of the best chemical defences in the animal world. They use an array of these defences, ranging from jets of boiling caustic fluids, paralysing toxins, and foul-smelling liquids to potent poisons that can cause immense harm. Chemical defence is commonly accompanied by a distinctive colouration or behavioural pattern that serves as a warning to the predators.

🐾 Borrowed Threads

Sea slugs lack any form of armour like shells, claws, or spines, but they are rarely bothered by even the hungriest of fish. The secret lies in the projections that cover their bodies. Many of these projections contain cnidocytes or stinging cells, which give off a barbed, poison-tipped thread the moment anything touches them.

Sea slugs themselves do not produce this poison. They retain it from their prey, the sea anemone. When sea slugs eat the sea anemones, the stinging cells from the latter's tentacles are not digested. These are transported by the slugs to the projections on their bodies and stored to be used in defence.

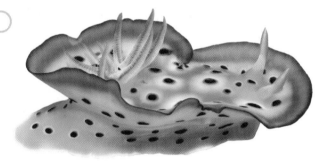

▲ *The bright colours of a sea slug serve as the first warning to its predators*

🐾 Velvety Smarts

Onychophorans, also known as velvet worms, live in tropical regions. These are known to squirt an odourless fluid from the glands on the ends of the projections on their heads. It can be squirted from a distance of almost 15 centimetres. The fluid then hardens immediately, disabling the predator.

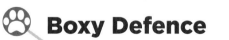

◀ *Velvet worms have been around for over 500 million years*

🐾 Whiplash

A whip scorpion raises its abdomen when it senses danger, and releases an acidic spray on its predator, which it dispels from its large glands.

◀ *Whip scorpions do not have tails. They resemble spiders*

🐾 Boxy Defence

Box jellyfish are named so because of the box-like appearance of their heads. These are transparent blue in colour. The poison of the box jellyfish is considered to be one of the deadliest in nature. It affects the heart, nervous system, as well as skin. It is fatal not just to animals but to human beings as well. If attacked, the victim undergoes intense pain and could die of heart failure. If the victim does survive, the pain can last for months.

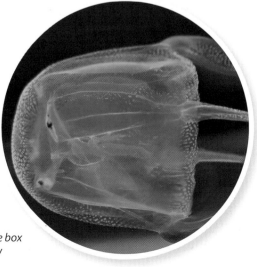

▶ *The venom released by the box jellyfish can even stun its prey*

Migratory Invertebrates

Marine invertebrates either migrate voluntarily or are swept away by strong ocean currents. Migration is the seasonal movement that relocates the invertebrates from one location to another for reasons including weather, food, and reproduction. Invertebrates end up covering a large distance during this time.

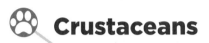 Planktonic Organisms

Planktons become aquatic drifters as they are carried forward by ocean currents. They travel vertically in a fixed rhythm. During the night, microscopic planktonic organisms travel in the upper waters and are followed by their predators—the fish. They are also relocated by pelagic birds who live in the open sea and prey on plankton and other plants. Planktons usually remain embedded in the bottom of the ocean during the day and come out at dusk.

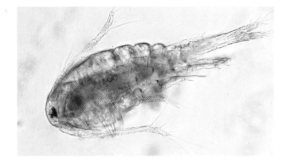
▲ *Freshwater aquatic zooplankton rely on ocean currents to migrate*

Crustaceans

Crustaceans migrate the farthest, especially during their reproductive cycle. Some travel even as far as 240 kilometres! Female crabs, for instance, mate and lay their eggs on the shore before returning to the depths of the ocean.

Some crabs have adapted to land and migrate to the water for the purpose of reproduction. The robber crabs are a classic example of this phenomenon as they return to land right after they finish laying their eggs and are followed back by their young after they have hatched.

The Chinese crabs, among other freshwater crabs, remain in the water for 4–5 years, migrating to brackish waters solely to lay eggs. Their young spend a year in these waters, before migrating back to freshwater.

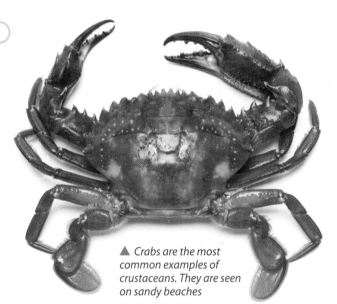
▲ *Crabs are the most common examples of crustaceans. They are seen on sandy beaches*

☀ Isn't It Amazing!

There are more than 45,000 species of crustaceans that live in different coastal environments. Among them are the amazing crabs which can live in salt water, freshwater, and even brackish waters. There are two broad categories of crabs: land crabs and sea crabs. But even land crabs need to spend some time in the water. In water, crabs breathe with their gills which are in cavities under the sides of the carapace. In land crabs, these cavities are much larger and modified to act as lungs.

Seasonal Migration

In the winter, clam worms live among algae and rock crevices. In the summer, they become planktonic and migrate a far distance from the coastal waters in Europe. There, they carry out the process of reproduction. Near Fiji and the South Pacific, the palolo worms develop reproductive cells in the posterior segments. In the months of October and November, the worms live among coral reefs until they shed off their genital cells and rise to the surface of the waters.

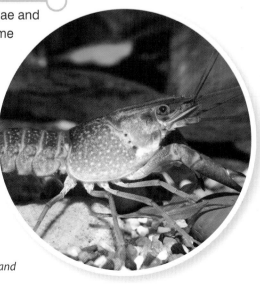
▶ *The painted crayfish is a benthic species. It lives and even migrates across the bottom of the ocean*

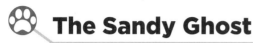

Clever Camouflage

Camouflage means to blend in the surroundings. Invertebrates use different methods of camouflage while waiting for a prey or while hiding from a predator. Many animals have been using this tactic for millions of years. They are impressive in their array of colours and patterns. Invertebrates might be tough, and they may possess chemical weapons, but in the big bad world, being small creatures, many need to use camouflage to survive.

🐾 The Sandy Ghost

Ghost crabs blend well in the sand dunes that are available in plenty on the beaches that they inhabit. The word 'ghost' in their name refers to the fact that these crabs can quickly disappear from sight using their six strong legs. They use camouflage well and lie in wait on the beach, with just two eyes protruding out. The moment a prey such as other crabs, lizards, insects, or clams approach them, the ghost crabs grab and devour it. To hide from the predator, ghost crabs simply vanish into their small burrows.

▲ *Ghost crabs are also known as sand crabs*

🐾 Light Play

Cuttlefish belong to the mollusc family. They have eight arms and two tentacles which are used to capture the prey. The cuttlefish have the amazing ability to change colour within seconds. They do it with the help of pigmented organs called chromatophores. The invertebrate expands or contracts these chromatophores, creating an array of colours. The colour-changing property of the cuttlefish is one of the best camouflage techniques on the planet.

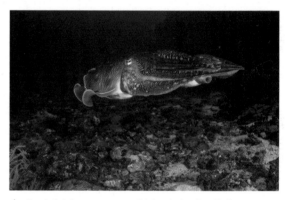

▲ *Cuttlefish have venom which can be deadly for human beings*

🐾 Deadly Golden Touch

The goldenrod crab spider, or flower spider, can blend in with a range of flowers by changing its colour. This change of colour from white to yellow takes about three weeks; the reverse takes six days. The spider sits in wait for an innocent prey on the flower, grabs it with its front legs, and kills it with its venom.

🐾 Hidden Beauty

Oregonia gracilis is found in the north-western coasts of the USA and Japan. It is also called the decorator crab and has a graceful appearance. Using its front legs, the crab picks up algae, sponges, wood chips, and any other marine detritus. The fragments are then modified by the crab using its mouth.

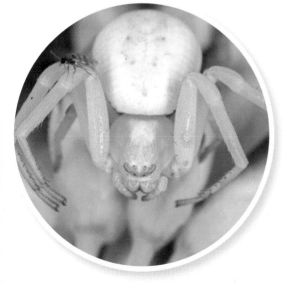

▲ *The goldenrod crab spider often sits on goldenrod flowers or daisies which are white or yellow in colour*

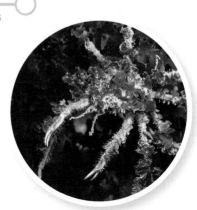

▶ *Sometimes a decorator crab looks like a moving rock. It camouflages itself with different items, which is why it has been given the name 'decorator'*

Hearty Meals

Like all other beings, invertebrates too need to eat to survive. They have a varied diet as some prefer to eat only plants, while others are voracious carnivores. Some are even fiercer carnivores than lions, tigers and wolves. Some invertebrates are decomposers, which means that they feed on dead plants and animals. Few are omnivores, which means that they eat plants as well as animals.

Aristotle's Lantern

The common sea urchin is an omnivore. Like the name suggests, it lives in the sea and eats algae, seaweed as well as mussels and barnacles. This animal feeds by means of a complex structure called Aristotle's lantern. Five plates made of calcified materials surround the mouth and come together as a beak. The sea urchin uses this beak to scrape off algae from the rocks. Scraping causes wear and tear of the plates, but the sea urchin has the ability of growing them back. Its mouth is located on the lower part of its body, while the anus is at the top. It has got a powerful bite, strong enough to eat the toughest of seaweeds.

▲ Some species of sea urchins have venomous spines on their bodies that are harmful to human beings

The Giant Crawl

Scolopendra gigantea is the world's largest centipede, reaching the length of almost 30 centimetres. The invertebrate is found in Central America and parts of South America. All centipedes are carnivores, but these can even immobilise and hold small vertebrates such as mice, frogs, small birds and bats using their poisonous forcipules, which are venom-filled sharp claws. Apart from vertebrates, the *Scolopendra gigantea* eats insects, spiders, snails and worms.

They have 21–23 pairs of legs and spiny rear legs with which they can attack their predators. They are nocturnal creatures with poor eyesight, but their antennae help them sense the prey. *Scolopendra gigantea* have numerous spiracles or respiratory openings; due to these openings, the creatures can lose water, leading to dehydration. To avoid this fate, they live in moist areas.

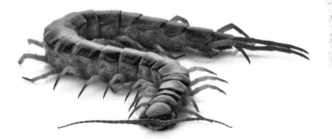

▲ *Scolopendra gigantea can refer to the Peruvian giant yellow-leg centipede or the Amazon giant centipede*

▶ *Dung beetles are decomposers*

Dung Eaters

Dung beetles are one tough species. As the name suggests, they primarily survive on dung of animals such as cattle and sheep; however, there are also a few who eat decomposing leaves and other rotting matter. The larvae eat solid dung, while the adults suck out nutrition from the dung ball.

In Australia, the native dung beetles have been known to feed on kangaroo dung but find it difficult to decompose dung from cattle and sheep. Australia has a large number of both of these animals; hence the breakdown of their faeces became an issue. So, African and European dung beetles were introduced in Australia in order to tackle the same.

The Ancient Sponges

Sea sponges are ancient animals with a basic structure. They evolved about 500 million years ago and have outlived the dinosaurs. These simple animals live in the seas, in shallow waters, as well as in the depths of the ocean, as deep as 8,500 metres. You will rarely find a floating sponge; these are seen attached to rocks, sand, or mud. There are close to 5,000 species of sponges in the world.

 ## Primitive Sponge

Sponges are animals with no organs. They have no eyes, legs, blood, heart, or brain. They are made of cells and fibres, which form the outer lining, surrounding a central cavity. The most important part of the sponge is its pores. It is through these pores that water moves in and out, filtering out the food needed for its existence, removing waste materials, and supplying the animal with oxygen.

 ## Diet

Sponges eat microorganisms, seaweed, animal eggs, larvae, and even small crustaceans such as barnacles and crabs.

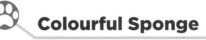 ## Colourful Sponge

Sponges can range from a size of 0.5 centimetres to almost 6 feet in height. A sponge discovered in Hawaii in recent times is as large as a minivan. It is almost 12 feet long and 7 feet wide.

Some species of sponges are shapeless, while there are others with a distinct shape. Tubular or vase sponges have structures like chimneys that create air currents to suck water into their feeding chambers. Some other species, such as the sea orange, have a spherical shape, while others may be shaped like cups or fans.

Deep-water dwelling sponges have a dull appearance, while those living in shallow waters come in an array of colours ranging from violet, blue, pink, red, and yellow to even black. Few sponges appear green because of the green algae residing in them. Algae and sponges share a symbiotic relationship, which means they are mutually helpful to each other. The algae find their homes in sponges, while the sponges get nutrition from them.

◄ *These large green organisms are called brain corals. Their name is inspired by the several deep grooves on the surface that resemble the grooves in human brains*

Reproduction

To create the next generation, some sponges grow buds, which break away from the main body and grow into new sponges; while others are hermaphrodites, which means that they have both male and female germ cells in them, which are brought together to create larvae.

The larvae swim away from the primary sponge. They float around for a few hours or days, until they find an attachment, where they grow into new adult sponges. Sponges can live for a year based on the environmental conditions of their surroundings. Few are known to live for several years. Sponges could at times be attacked by disease of which not much is known.

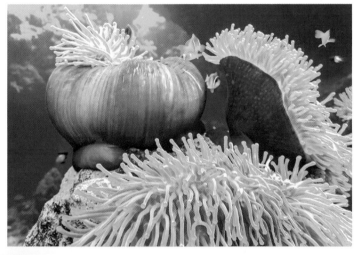

▲ Sponges are filter-feeders which means they capture microbes from the water that passes through their pores

Spikes and Pokes

Some sponges are smooth in appearance, while others have projections called spicules. These are rough, hard, and sharp. They are made of substances such as lime or chalk. They don't just give firmness to the body of a sponge, but also help keep away predators.

In Real Life

In ancient Greece and Rome, sponges were used to apply paint or as mops. Now they are used in surgical medicine, painting, pottery, decoration and even for bathing. The best sponges are found in the Mediterranean Sea. They have been gathered so extensively that the population has declined rapidly. It is said it will take years for it to grow back. Due to the restrictions put by governments, sponges cannot be taken from the wild anymore. They are commercially grown in various parts of the world.

Defence

Most sponges need saltwater to survive. However, there are a few which grow in brackish water while members of the *Spongillidae* family live in freshwaters. Sponges cannot bear to be in the open air for long. If air fills up in their pores, they wither away.

Some types of snails, slugs, crabs, and fish eat sponges. Not too many animals like to make sponges their food because of their disagreeable smell as well as taste. This is why the hermit crab is smart. It makes the sponge its home. Predators such as fish stay away from these unpleasant sponges, so the crab leads a protected life.

▶ Tube sponges thrive best in areas with strong currents

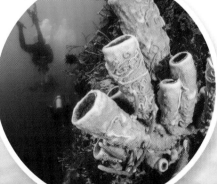

The Colourful Corals

There are almost 5,000 species of corals found in the world. Like sponges, these are ancient animals, having existed for almost 500 million years. The individual organism is called a polyp, which can survive on its own, but prefers to live in colonies called coral reefs. Corals cannot grow in freshwater, so they live in the salty seas.

Coral Polyp Interior

Coral polyps are tiny animals resembling sea anemones. Their base is a hard structure made of calcium carbonate, also called limestone. It is called the calicle. This is the basic structure of a coral reef.

The coral **polyp** resembles a vase filled with flowers. The mouth of the polyp is the only opening present. It takes in food and also removes waste. It is surrounded by tubular tentacles, which are covered with nematocytes or stinging cells. These are used for defence or to sting a prey. Also, they help the mouth carry out its functions.

The polyp is covered with an outer epidermis layer and an inner gastrodermis layer. Between the two is mesoglea, a jelly-like substance, which acts as a **hydrostatic** skeleton. The stomach is made up of digestive filaments, which aid in digestion. Individual polyps are connected with one another by a small filament of living tissue called coenosarc.

Nematocyst · Outer epidermis · Tentacle · Mouth · Mesoglea · Digestive Filament · Stomach · Septum · Gastrodermis · Coenosarc · Theca · Basal plate

▲ *The average polyp can be 1–3 millimetres in diameter*

A Dash of Colour

Did you know a coral polyp is actually transparent? Then how are the reefs so colourful? Inside the coral live tiny colourful algae called zooxanthellae. They impart vibrant and colourful shades to the reefs. Corals and algae share a symbiotic relationship. While corals offer homes to the algae, algae absorb waste in the form of carbon dioxide and phosphates and provide the corals with the essential oxygen and other by-products of photosynthesis. Corals are known to eat plankton and small fish.

Beautiful Creation

Once a year, after a full moon, when the water temperature is correct, the entire colony of corals produces male and female gametes, or germ cells. It is a spectacular sight, with cascades of small, tiny specks floating in the water. The male and female gametes come together to create small larvae called planula. These larvae float in the water for a short time, before they embed themselves on rocks. If the conditions are right, a coral colony formation begins, which grows at a rate of 4 inches per year.

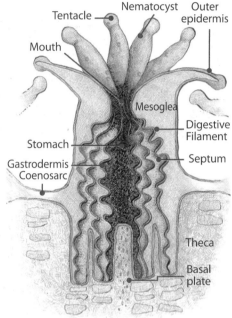

▶ *Due to the effects of global warming, coral reefs are dying off. Some species of corals have become threatened. Scientists are working hard to restore coral reefs using various techniques like coral farming, reattaching broken coral pieces, etc*

In Real Life

The best place in the world to see the coral reefs is the Great Barrier Reef off the coast of eastern Australia. Almost the size of Japan, it is home to innumerable species of sea turtles, whales, dolphins, sea snakes and almost 10 per cent of the world's total fish species.

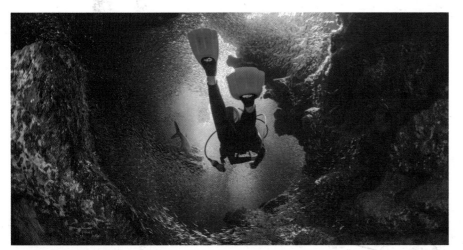

Isn't It Amazing!

Do you know why corals are found in shallow, warm tropical waters? It is so that the Sun's rays penetrate deep enough to help algae with photosynthesis, a reaction necessary for the existence of corals. Coral reefs should remain healthy for a balanced environment.

▲ *Coral reefs are known as the "rainforests of the sea"*

A Complete Life

When a coral polyp dies out, a new polyp uses the remains as a base to attach itself to the reef. In this way, the reef keeps expanding, creating an ecosystem that supports more than 25 per cent of marine life. The reefs provide animals with safe places to live, hide, and find food.

Today, coral reefs are threatened by pollution and global warming. When they feel stressed due to environmental changes, they simply expel their resident algae. This is when the reef looks bleached. If the stress is not reversed, the colony starts to die out. In many parts of the world, corals are reaching this fate and sadly, it spells doom for many species that thrive in this fragile ecosystem.

Scientists are trying to reverse the effects of global warming on coral reefs by reattaching the coral pieces to the reefs. Scuba divers are further trained to work on restoration projects. They attach new pieces of corals to the reefs using a type of cement. This gives the coral reef another chance for survival.

▼ *Fish and other living species rely on coral reefs for food, shelter, and protection from predators*

Parasitic Invertebrates

Living inside another plant or animal can be a good source of nutrition. This is exactly what parasites do to have their needs met. A parasite lives inside a host without a symbiotic relationship. The host provides the parasite with food, water, and shelter. In return, the parasite might harm the host or simply live without causing major issues.

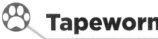 Tapeworms

Tapeworms are flat, segmented, and can parasitise the digestive tracts of many vertebrate species, including human beings. The largest of the tapeworms live in sperm whales and can grow to almost 100 feet. In human beings, tapeworms can be as long as 60 feet.

Adult Stage

An adult tapeworm living in the human gut has a head or a scolex which attaches to the gut wall, and suckers and a tail of hundreds of identical segments or proglottids. A tapeworm has no intestine and absorbs nourishment through its surface.

Lifecycle

Mature segments carrying tapeworm eggs break off from the tail and are excreted as faeces by the host. Many times it happens that the infected segments are eaten by cattle or pigs while taking in their food. The eggs enter the animal's intestine. Intestinal **enzymes** in the gut breakdown the eggshells. The eggs penetrate the intestinal wall and through the bloodstream are carried to the muscles where they develop into larvae. These larvae are called oncospheres.

If a human being happens to eat undercooked pig or cattle meat carrying the tapeworm, he or she is infected. The worm attaches itself to the human gut once more and the cycle is repeated. There are 54 species of tapeworms which can infect human beings.

Threat to People

Most often tapeworms cause weight loss, abdominal pain, loss of appetite, diarrhoea, and weakness in human beings. In rare cases, they may lead to intestinal blockage. In this case, the doctor gives a course of medicine to clear out the infection.

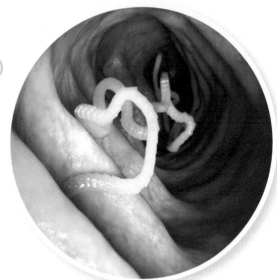

▲ *Tapeworms are caused due to the intake of contaminated food or water*

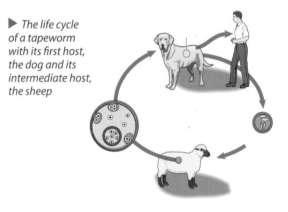

▶ *The life cycle of a tapeworm with its first host, the dog and its intermediate host, the sheep*

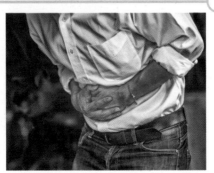

▲ *Adult tapeworms can live up to 30 years in a host*

⊙ Incredible Individuals

Before the 17th century, it was a little difficult to learn about diseases caused by tapeworms as most people could not differentiate between the various tapeworm species. By the 17th century, people knew that there were two distinct and separate types. It was Felix Plater (1536–1614), a physician from Switzerland, who described the two tapeworms—*Diphyllobothrium latum* and *Taenia*. Plater overcame several obstacles to complete his studies as he grew up at a time when religious persecution terrorised his country. After completing his studies, he became a physician and professor of medicine. He also studied anatomy, making several important discoveries in the field.

A Rounded Existence

Nematodes, also known as roundworms, are one of the most abundant animals on Earth. They have a range of habitats and can live as parasites in plants, animals and human beings. They live in soil, freshwater, marine environments and even in items such as vinegar and beer. Close to 20,000 identified species exist. However, there could be more in number according to scientists. Roundworms come in a range of sizes, right from the microscopic variety to ones that are as long as 23 feet.

In Real Life

Ascaris lumbricoides is a parasitic roundworm which causes infection in human beings. The infection is common in warm tropical regions. The *ascaris lumbricoides* can grow to a size of 35 centimetres! If the host carries both male and female worms, on fertilisation, a female can lay more than 200,000 fertilised eggs per day.

Elephantiasis

The filarial worm, belonging to the phyla nematode, causes elephantiasis. This is an unpleasant tropical disease. The victim's affected body parts, mainly the legs, swell up to gigantic proportions. The filarial worm needs two hosts. One is the mosquito; it is in the mosquito's body that the worm completes its larval phase. Once the mosquito bites human beings, it diffuses the larvae into the human body. The larvae complete their journey to adulthood in the lymphatic system. Once here, they block the system, leading to swelling of tissues and further weaken the affected body part.

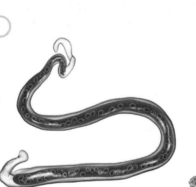

▲ Tiny filarial worms lead to big swellings

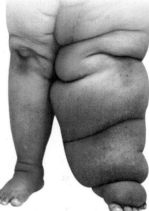

▲ The legs of a person suffering from elephantiasis shown for comparison

The Oak Apples

Hard, round marble galls, also called oak apples are commonly seen on oak trees. It is the tree's response to an infection caused by a parasitic insect called the gall wasp. The female lays eggs on the tissues of leaves or twigs of the oak tree. When the eggs hatch, the tissues around the larvae, also called grubs, swell up, creating gall. When the grub leaves the gall, it creates a hole. Most often, the affected twig or leaf is shed off by the tree. In general, galls do not affect the life of an oak tree, unless there are numerous ones on the bark as well.

▲ Marble galls "are caused by a tiny wasp called Andricus kollari

▶ The gall wasps are sometimes incorrectly called gallflies

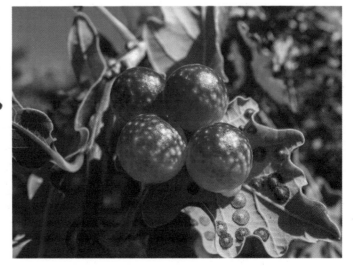

▲ Oak apples are sponge-like and spherical in shape.

The Slimy Snails

Phylum Mollusca is truly a diverse world consisting of more than 100,000 species which reside in marine, freshwater, and terrestrial environments. Of these, commonly seen are snails, the slow creatures which inhabit almost all gardens in the world, especially after heavy rainfall.

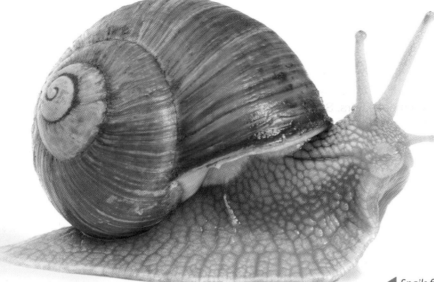

🐾 Habitat

Apart from gardens, snails live in oceans, freshwater lakes, ponds, rivers, and on land. When they are on land, snails are found in dark places such as rock crevices and wood logs. Many live near water sources, as they need to keep themselves moist. This is because, like amphibians, snails have thin skin which does not retain moisture.

◀ *Snails first evolved 500 million years ago*

🐾 Snail Trail

Have you seen a snail moving? If so, you might have noticed a trail of something wet that it leaves behind on its path. This is the slime released by the animal to move forward with minimum friction. Also, snails use their slime in harsh weather conditions, such as summers and winters. They seal the shell entrance with slime, which hardens and acts like a door that protects the animal inside. In conducive weather conditions, the slime plug is broken, and the snail moves about freely.

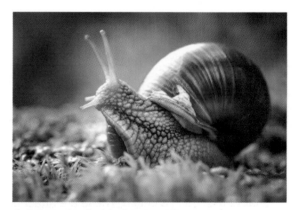

▲ *Salt can fatally dehydrate a snail*

🐾 Protection

Snails need to protect themselves from predators. How do they do it? They have a shell made up of calcium carbonate. This protects their internal organs. The interesting feature about the shell is its spiral structure. Also, snails have an organ called the operculum. It is like a flap; the moment the invertebrate senses danger, it retreats into the shell, pulling the flap over the opening.

▶ *The rings on a snail's shell indicate its age*

👪 In Real Life

> Apart from snails, oysters, clams, mussels, scallops, squids, and winkles are a few molluscs eaten around the world. They are an important source of food for people living in coastal regions. The practice of snail harvesting has led to many of their species being put on the endangered list of animals.

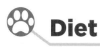 Snail Senses

These invertebrates have four tentacles. The two lower ones are used to smell, while the two upper ones are sensory, which means they help them feel. The upper tentacles often have two eyes at the ends. These tentacles can be retracted completely.

Diet

A snail's tongue has many teeth; they are called radula and there can be thousands of them. These help snails chop through algae and plants sticking to rocks. Few larger snails are meat eaters. Snails that are decomposers are friends to human beings. They help in breaking down dead plant and animal material; and the soil regains its nutrients, making farmers happy. Snails are also used in a French delicacy called escargot, which is popular all over the world. The name literally means 'edible snail'.

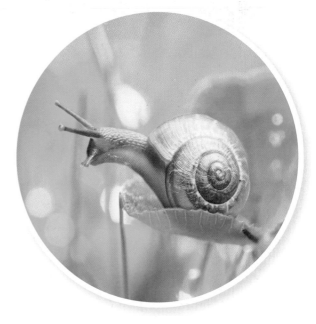

▲ *All land snails have the ability to retract their tentacles*

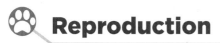 Powelliphanta

Powelliphanta are large snails, with an oversized shell in a hue of colours such as red, yellow, black, and brown. These snails live in the grasslands and forests of New Zealand. They are carnivores. They love earthworms in particular and also eat slugs.

Reproduction

Different snails reproduce in different ways. Some are **hermaphrodites**, which means they are male and female at the same time. Many of these snails do not need a partner to produce babies. Some snails need a partner even if they are hermaphrodites. Some other snail species have distinct male and female members.

Snails lay eggs in a clutch. These are attached to a wood log, tree, or ground. In water, snail eggs attach themselves to rock surfaces. They are covered with a jelly to prevent them from drying. Each clutch can have a few to as many as 600 eggs. The Chinese mystery snail can lay almost 100 eggs, while Ramshorn snails lay only about 10–12 eggs.

Isn't It Amazing!

Most molluscs have a large and strong muscular foot. It is this foot that helps these animals move, dig, attach, and capture prey. Snails are gastropods or 'stomach-footed', which means that their muscular foot is on the lower part of their body, near the stomach.

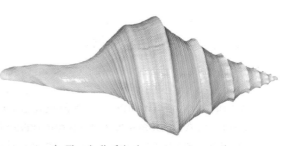

▲ *The shell of the largest marine snail, the Australian trumpet, can grow to almost 2 ft in length*

▼ *The African giant snail is the largest land snail in the world with a shell that is 10.75 in long*

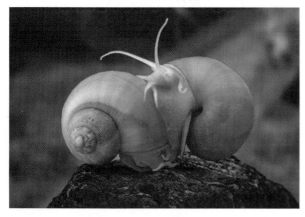

▲ *The spike-topped apple snails are large freshwater snails from South America with a shell diameter as big as 8 centimetres*

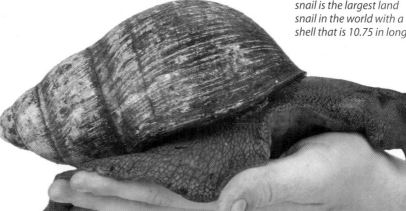

Meet the Squids

Squids belong to the family of the elusive cephalopods that also includes octopuses and cuttlefish. The ten-armed cephalopods are a part of the order Teuthoidea and are abundant in both coastal and ocean waters. They have short heads and long tubular bodies.

Body

The 10 arms of the squids have diverse features to help their survival. Two of these arms are slender tentacles and the rest are toothed, brisk rings that they use for suction. Their bodies are protected by a sharp internal shell. They have very distinct eyes located on the sides of their head, and excellent vision. Some species of squids are swift swimmers whereas some attach themselves to plankton for movement. Squids usually eat small crabs and fish. They are eaten by whales, bony fish, and human beings.

▼ *There are several species of squids in the oceans. Below is an example of the hooked squid*

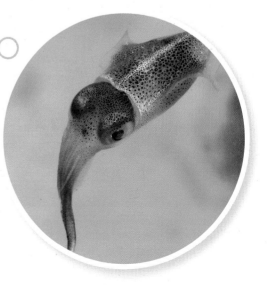

The Flying Squid

There have been many sightings of squids who are airborne. Scientists have always known of their gliding abilities, but numerous recent sightings indicate that some species of squids actively 'fly'. So, referring to the act as gliding may underrepresent this agile airborne quality.

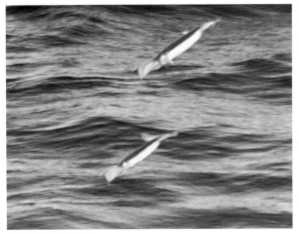

▲ *Japanese flying squid*

These flying squids flap their fins like wings and flare their tentacles in a radial pattern, as if controlling their trajectories. Squids thrust themselves above water by a process called jet propulsion. They have a soft mantle that soaks up water. They also have a flexible tube right below their head that shoots out this water. By adjusting the direction of the tube, they determine the direction of their flight. They use this technique underwater to feast on prey and escape predators. However, in more recent times, squids have been seen using this ability to fly above water as well. Some squids also swim backwards by spreading their tentacles in a web-like fashion. Scientists have spotted squids using this technique to stop or slow down even as they fly.

Exploding Populations

Squids have fast-paced lives. They live only for a year and lay many eggs that mature rapidly. Their young have low mortality rates because their eggs are covered with a protective layer. However, scientists have tracked a change in the lifecycle of the squids because of climate change. The Humboldt squids previously weighed 1 to 2 kg and followed the one-year life cycle. But now they thrive in the warm waters of the eastern Pacific. The winters have been getting colder, resulting in a longer maturity cycle for these squids. They end up growing extremely large in size.

Changing Colours

Squids are skilled at changing their colours just like chameleons and octopuses. They do it to camouflage and hide from potential predators. They can also glow brightly. Squids have two special groups of pigment cells called chromatophores and photophores present in their skin. Chromatophores are controlled by muscular contractions. By modifying the size of these cells, squids can change the colour of their bodies. They have powerful eyesight that can detect both intensity and colour of different lights. They use this feature to mirror the colour of the ocean floor or any landscape they want to blend in with.

Squids change colours in order to threaten or warn the prey as well as to hide from their predators. With the chromatophore cells, squids produce an intense light by the process of bioluminescence. This happens because of combustion between luciferin, oxygen, and the enzyme luciferase. By the end of this reaction, the organism typically emits a blue-green glow. This light can be used for many functions, one of them being communication.

▲ A glowing purpleback squid that naturally changes colour in the ocean. It also changes to a bright pink

Incredible Individuals

Tsunemi Kubodera is a zoologist from Japan. In 2004, he managed to capture a photograph of the giant squid in its natural habitat with his team. He was then able to record the giant squid on film. Both times he captured an adult and live giant squid. He also managed to film the animal in its natural habitat. He was the first to do all this, but it was not easy finding the elusive giant squid.

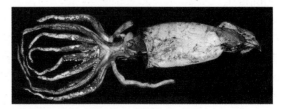

▲ A specimen of the giant squid. It measures four metres, excluding its tentacles

Elusive Giants

Giant squids are the largest ones on record. They grow to 13 metres in length. Some giant squids are 900 kilograms in weight. Though they are so huge, scientists have a hard time finding them because they live deep underwater. They are studied using their dead bodies that float to the surface.

The Friendly Earthworms

Worms are so varied and numerous across the world that they form different groups. One such group is the annelids. Their elongated bodies are divided into numerous ring-like segments. They are found in oceans, burrowing in land, or even attaching themselves to the host as blood suckers. There are over 9,000 identified species of these worms in the world today.

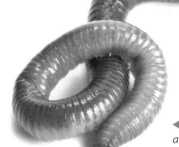

◄ Earthworms are also known as angleworms

Habitat

Earthworms are native to Europe. However, they are found in big numbers in North America as well as western Asia. They do not live in the desert regions or areas with permanent snow coverage as such conditions do not suit them.

Burrowed Life

The annuli or the segments of the earthworm are covered with small bristles called setae, which help the earthworm move. The average length of the earthworm might be 7–9 centimetres, but it can burrow almost up to 6.5 feet deep into the soil. It can burrow all day, and crawl above to feed at night.

Diet

The mouth of the earthworm is at its first segment. They eat soil, taking in nutrients from the dead leaves and roots. A single earthworm can eat almost one-third its body weight. The remains are excreted as casts. It is the highly nutritious cast that transports minerals and other vital nutrients to the surface of the soil, making it richer for the plants growing in it. Through their burrowing, the worms aerate the soil. No wonder this small animal is a friend to the farmers.

Reproduction

Earthworms are hermaphrodites, which means a single animal will have both male and female parts. But they do not self-fertilise. They need another earthworm to create the next generation.

The main part through which the exchange of sex cells takes place is the saddle or the clitellum. It is seen as a bulge with several enlarged segments. It is through this that the earthworms exchange the sperms or the male cells to fertilise the egg cells. On mating, each worm forms a small cocoon using the liquid secreted by the clitellum. It is in this that the exchanged cells are stored. The cocoon slips off the body of the earthworm and is buried in the soil. In two to four weeks, small baby earthworms are born.

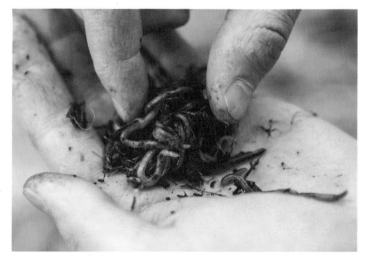

▲ Baby earthworms pulled from the earth

◄ Earthworms do not have eyes, but they can sense light

The Bloodthirsty Leeches

Leeches are slightly flat-looking worms. These muscular worms can lengthen and shorten their bodies as desired. They have 34 segments on their bodies along with suckers, which distinguish them from other worms. The suckers are present at both ends—a small one at the front and a large one at the posterior end. Leeches can be small or big. The giant Amazon leech can grow almost up to 45 centimetres in length.

Quest for Survival

Some leeches prey on small worms, insect larvae, and snails. The horse leech can grow up to 16 centimetres long and swallow its food whole. Other leeches are parasites. They live on the bodily fluids of other animals.

The leech clamps itself onto other animals. It then uses its three sets of tiny teeth to make its way into the skin. It sucks blood and other bodily fluids up to almost five times its weight. The giant Amazon leech uses its six-inch long proboscis as a needle to suck blood from the host. A leech can survive for weeks before needing another feed. This is because there is a pouch in its digestive system where it can store the food that it eats for weeks or even months. So, leeches do not need to find food very often.

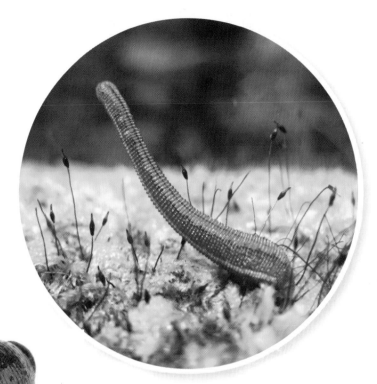

▲ Each leech has: 10 eyes, 6 hearts, 10 pouches for storing blood, 32 brains, and 200 enzymes

▲ The bodies of leeches are segmented. Notice the 34 segments on this leech's body

Usefulness

Leeches can suck blood from their host and make it weak. They also attach themselves to human beings. The use of leeches in therapy or treatment is called 'leech therapy'. This was very common before modern medical practices evolved. Doctors used leeches to increase blood circulation and break down blood clots.

There is a species called the European medicinal leech. It is now used to prevent blood clots in human beings during surgery. There is a substance extracted from the tissue of the leech's body called anticoagulant hirudin which is used for the purpose of preventing blood clots. Apart from this, the saliva in leeches contains substances that can anesthetise wounds. Also, substances from the Amazonian leeches are used to dissolve blood clots.

In Real Life

The bright red tubifex is also called a bloodworm because of its colour. The colour is due to the presence of haemoglobin, a pigment known for its affinity to oxygen. It is the same pigment present in human beings. It takes oxygen from the water and transports it through the skin of the worm. The pigment is so abundant that the bloodworm can even stay in stagnant water with very low oxygen content. In general, these worms are found in freshwater. Some of them are also brown or tan in colour.

▶ In the older days, when a patient had his fingers re-attached, he might have had to use leech therapy to prevent blood build-up

Crabs & Other Crustaceans

Crustaceans belong to the arthropod group. Crabs, lobsters, shrimps, and prawns are common examples of crustaceans. They have tough, calcareous exoskeletons. They also have two pairs of appendages in front of the mouth and paired appendages near the mouth which function as jaws. There exist about 45,000 species of crustaceans across the world. Most of these are aquatic in nature.

Crabby Behaviour

When we talk about crustaceans, the most common one that comes to mind is the crab. Crabs are a delicacy around the world. A typical crab has a hard, shell-like cover with a small abdomen tucked inside it. It has five pairs of limbs. One pair consists of large pincers and four pairs consist of the limbs used for walking. Crabs live in sea water, but there are exceptions which live in rivers and lakes.

▲ *The stone crab can regenerate its claws if they are removed*

Out of the Blue

The blue crab has a tint of sapphire blue in its claws. This is where it gets its name from. The female blue crab has bright orange tips on her claws. Its shell is brownish in colour. It is found around coastal waters right from Nova Scotia till Uruguay. The crab is an omnivore, which means it eats both plants as well as meat. It eats mussels, smaller blue crabs, snails, fish, and even carrion.

Large male crabs can have a shell width of almost 22 centimetres. These crabs are excellent swimmers because they use their paddle-shaped hind appendages to swim. They are known for their sweet meat because of which they are harvested in large numbers. Unfortunately, since they are sensitive to the environment and climatic changes, their numbers are on the decline.

Baby Boom

Blue crabs, like other hard-shelled crustaceans, mate only after the female has moulted. Yes, most crabs moult, which means they shed their exoskeleton to regrow a new one. Mating occurs when the new shell is soft. The male protects the female in this exposed, vulnerable stage. The female blue crab lays eggs which she carries around with her. The eggs are held in place under the abdomen, with the help of firm bristles. In this stage, she is said to be 'in berry'.

When the eggs are ready to hatch, they are released as larvae. The transparent 'zoea', as the first baby stage is called, is about two millimetres long and feeds on plankton. 'Megalopa' is the next stage, which is more crab-like. Finally, at the width of about 4 millimetres, the 'juvenile', or young adult is completely like a mature crab. It just has to grow in size.

▶ *Male blue crabs mate with multiple females over their lifespan*

◀ *Female blue crabs mate only once in their lives*

▲ *Male crabs are bigger than female crabs. Males have blue claws, while females have red-tipped claws*

Cousin of the Crab

Lobsters, like their crab cousins, are enjoyed as a delicacy, especially with butter and a squeeze of lime. These creatures live in varied habitats such as oceans, brackish waters, and freshwaters. Like crabs, lobsters have five pairs of appendages. While four pairs allow them to walk around, the remaining one forms the sharp pincers used to hold and crush the prey. The four walking leg pairs are attached to the thorax, which is the middle part of the lobster's body. The abdomen in the lobster is at the rear end, like a tail.

Lobsters cannot see properly, but they have a sharp sense of smell and taste. They use their long antennae for the same. They feed on shellfish, small fish, algae, and plankton.

This invertebrate is well-protected with a tough shell. The abdomen is covered with a series of plates. Lobsters are known to moult in order to grow. They can live for a long time, for almost 50 years. Their common abodes are rocks, sea grasses, and self-dug holes.

Similar to crabs, female lobsters carry their eggs under their abdomen. They do so for almost a year, before releasing them as larvae. Their larvae go through a series of stages before they grow into adults.

▲ *Most lobsters are nocturnal, scavenging marine animals. There are many species of lobsters; some of them are called true lobsters.*

Woodlice

Woodlice look like insects but are crustaceans. There are about 3,500 species of woodlice in the world and these are among the few crustaceans that live on land. These invertebrates have 14 legs and a thick exoskeleton. When they grow too big for the exoskeleton, they moult.

Woodlice have two antennae at the front end with which they sense their surroundings and two small outgrowths called uropods at the rear, which they need for navigation. Uropods also produce a chemical in some woodlice species. This chemical is used to ward off predators. Woodlice survive off of rotting plants, fungi, and their own excretory matter. They live in dark and damp places, on walls, and on decaying tree barks.

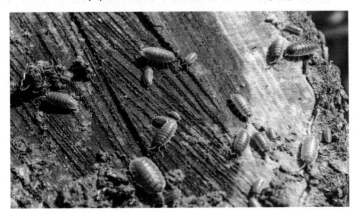

▲ *A close-up view of woodlice. The very first species of woodlice were marine species*

In Real Life

Coconut crabs, also known as robber crabs, are large crustaceans. An adult can reach the width of almost 100 centimetres and can weigh up to 4 kilograms. Their meat is a delicacy. These crabs live on land and in water. Using their sharp pincers, they climb trees near the shore and can break open coconuts.

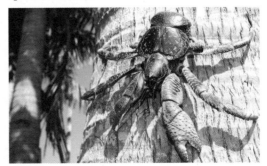

▲ *The claws of coconut crabs have the strongest pinch of any crustacean*

Creepy Crawlies

Spiders belong to an arthropod group called arachnids. The main feature of this group is that the animals here have 8 legs unlike crustaceans, which have 10 or more, while insects have 6 legs. Arachnids do not have wings or antennae. There are close to 80,000 species of arachnids spread across the world in a range of habitats, out of which more than 45,000 are spiders.

Appearance

The body of the spider is divided into two parts. The first part is the front cephalothorax, which consists of the spider's eyes, stomach, brain, glands that make poison, and mouth fangs. The second part is chelicerae or the spider's muscular jaws. It is the chelicerae that hold onto the prey while the spider injects it with poison.

Spiders cannot chew their food. Their fangs are like straws. They deliver enzymes into the prey, which make the prey mushy like a soup. Then they suck up the prey.

The spider also has leg-like pedipalps. These are not used for walking, but more as antennae to sense the objects that come in its way. It needs the pedipalps to hold its prey and even spin the legendary spiderweb.

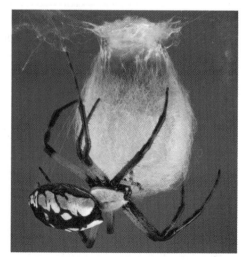
▲ The underside of a spider has thousands of silk glands that extrude silk through spinnerets

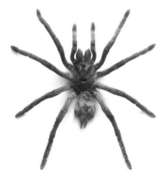

The back of the body is called the abdomen, which contains important internal organs. It is at the end of it that the silk-producing glands called spinnerets are present.

Spiders have a lot of hair on their legs. It is this hair which picks up vibrations and scents from the surroundings. Similar to other invertebrates, spiders have tough exoskeletons, which do not grow with them.

◀ Xenesthis immanis is a stunning spider with a star on its back

Silk Producers

Spiders make silk. It is this ability that sets them apart from other arthropods. They produce silk as a fluid containing a protein called fibroin. This solidifies into insoluble threads.

All spiders do not weave webs; instead many use the silk to spin protective cocoons around the eggs, to line their burrows and create a safety line (just in case they tumble). They also make these cocoons to wrap up their prey.

Spider silk is a strong, tenacious material. It is so strong that many spiders attach their silk thread to something, like the bark of a tree and use it to swing long distances. The spider's silk comes in different forms. The cocoon silk is delicate and soft, while the silk used to spin webs is sticky.

▲ An argiope spider building an egg case of silk after laying a yellow cluster of eggs

Webs

To spin a web, the spider needs some support like an anchor for the web's threads. This support could be rocks, vegetation, or any other solid surface. The spider selects a high perch and lets the thread travel until it touches and sticks to another object. More threads are spun, making a dense network.

Most webs are traps, but do not trap the spider itself. This is because it walks only on dry threads and uses special brushes on its claws to grip the threads. Spiders also release oil which forms a coating on their feet to prevent them from sticking to the web.

Spiderwebs could be in perfect geometric patterns or simply a mass of tangled threads. If the web is badly damaged, the spider can eat its own silk to reproduce it and make a new web.

The moment the prey touches the web, the silk wraps around it. The spiders release the poison using their fangs. Once the prey is paralysed, it is unwrapped and consumed.

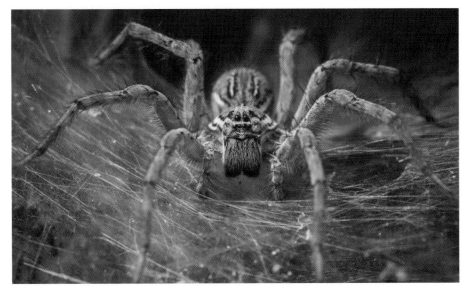

▲ Spiders have four pairs of eyes and, unlike other arthropods, have very keen vision

Isn't It Amazing!

The largest spider is the Goliath birdeater of South America. The body measures up to 13 centimetres, with a leg span of 30 centimetres. As the name suggests, it catches birds (although not very frequently), along with small mammals like mice, lizards, and other spiders as well.

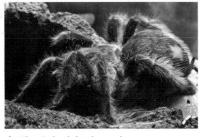

▲ The Goliath birdeater has an average weight of 175 grams

Poisonous Spiders

Though almost all spiders have poison, not all are harmful enough to hurt human beings. But there exist a few species of spiders with poison so powerful that they can harm most animals, including human beings. The black widow spider is a fierce arachnid, with its poison said to be deadlier than that of a rattlesnake. Its sting affects people too. If a human being is injected with the poison, they might have nausea, aches in their muscles, and breathing problems. The female black widow spider, after mating, at times eats the male spider. A close cousin, the brown widow spider, has poison twice as potent, but it is less aggressive.

◀ Black widow spider; widow spider nymphs are mostly white when they hatch from the egg sac

▶ Brazilian wandering spider; these spiders do not build webs and actively search for their prey

Setting a Trap

Trapdoor spiders live in burrows. Using their silk, they create a hinged door-like structure. The webbed door detects even the smallest of vibrations as a creature passes by. The silk in the web acts like a trap. Sometimes, the spider also lays long silk strands around the burrow which act like trap wires. The moment a creature touches the silk, the spider lying in wait, darts out of the burrow to inject it with its poison. It then drags the prey into the burrow, closing the trapdoor once more. Brazilian wandering spiders are considered to be the deadliest in the world. They not only use an aggressive defence position by raising their front legs in the air, but also have venom that is toxic even to the human nervous system. Their stings are said to be fatal on small children.

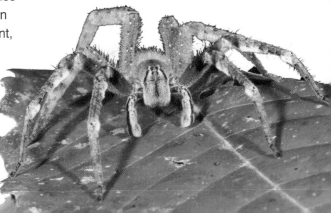

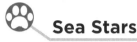

Star of the Show

The word echinoderm means 'hedgehog skin' in Greek and many of the species in this group are indeed spiny. These creatures live in the marine waters, so not many are familiar to us. But perhaps the most known and favourite is the starfish. In recent years the name starfish has been replaced with sea star, because the animal is technically not a fish.

Sea Stars

There are about 2,000 species of sea stars living in the warm and cold oceanic waters of the world. The most commonly known are the ones with five arms, but do you know there are species with as many as 40 arms? Underneath each arm, there are tiny tube-like feet which act as suction pumps, giving the sea star a unique adaptation that makes it capable of climbing vertical rocks. The arms have light-sensitive spots at the tips that help sea stars find food. These invertebrates have bony, spiny exoskeletons which protect them against their predators. Also, the bright colours act as a camouflage or a tool to ward off predators.

Regeneration

Sea stars have amazing regeneration skills. They can shed limbs in defence or to combat injury. The injured limb usually dies off. In its place, a new limb grows from the stump. Sometimes the new part is smaller than the original one. At other times, it branches into two, creating a six-limbed sea star.

Hunters

Sea stars are aggressive hunters. They feed on molluscs such as clams, mussels, oysters, and snails. They have an interesting technique to hunt down bivalve molluscs such as mussels. They grip the shell of mussels or similar creatures with their strong tube feet and keep pulling until the bivalve is exhausted and its shell opens.

▲ *Sea stars have no brain and no blood; they use filtered sea water to pump nutrients through their nervous system*

Diet

A sea star spills its stomach into the mouth of the prey. Enzymes from the sea star digest the prey, after which it is ingested by the animal. The stomach returns to its original place.

Crown-of-thorns Starfish

The crown-of-thorns starfish is an interesting invertebrate. It has up to 21 arms and these, along with the upper surface, have sharp, toxin-filled thorns that are 4 to 5 centimetres long. This sea star is a bane to the coral reefs. It can eat almost 10 square metres of coral reefs in one year. Also, a single female can produce close to 50 million eggs in one year. Australian coral reefs have suffered many an outbreak of crown-of-thorns, leading to massive destruction. Outbreaks of these starfish on coral reefs are often the result of overfishing, where the natural predator of the crown-of-thorns starfish is removed.

▲ *The crown-of-thorns starfish gets its name from the thorns that give it a biblical crown structure*

Breakaway

Brittle stars are cousins of the sea stars. They have close to 2,100 living species in the group. As the name suggests, the brittle star is indeed brittle. Parts of its long, delicate arms break off to regenerate soon. It has five arms radiating from a central disc. These arms can grow almost up to 2 ft in larger species. It uses its flexible arms to crawl across the sea floors.

Most brittle stars do not prefer the shallow tidal waters. They are found in deeper waters. Sometimes hundreds of brittle stars are found piled up on the sea floor. They feed on plankton, worms, and small molluscs. They also feed on the detritus, thus making them scavengers.

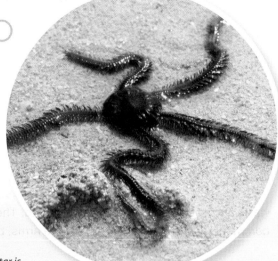

▶ *The brittle star is also called serpent star*

Like Feathers

Feather stars are also cousins of the sea star. They have 550 existing species. These invertebrates have feathery arms, which are used both for swimming and feeding. They use their legs called cirri to settle on corals, sponges, or any other perch in the sea. They move their long arms to capture edible material floating in water. Feather stars are commonly found in waters of the Indian Ocean right up to Japan.

Like the Lily

Similar to its namesake, the flower lily, sea lilies have a long stalk with which they attach themselves to the ocean. They have feathery arms that sway in the water. They may resemble a flower but are actually echinoderms. Most live in deep waters of the ocean, along the sea beds. They feed on detritus or floating edible particles. Other starfish also resemble the sea lily but they do not have the stalk, thus allowing them to be much more mobile than sea lilies.

▶ *Feather stars and sea lilies may look like plants, but they are related to starfish. All of them are echinoderms*

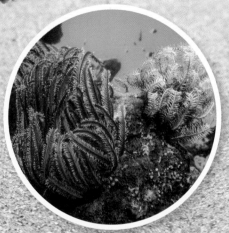

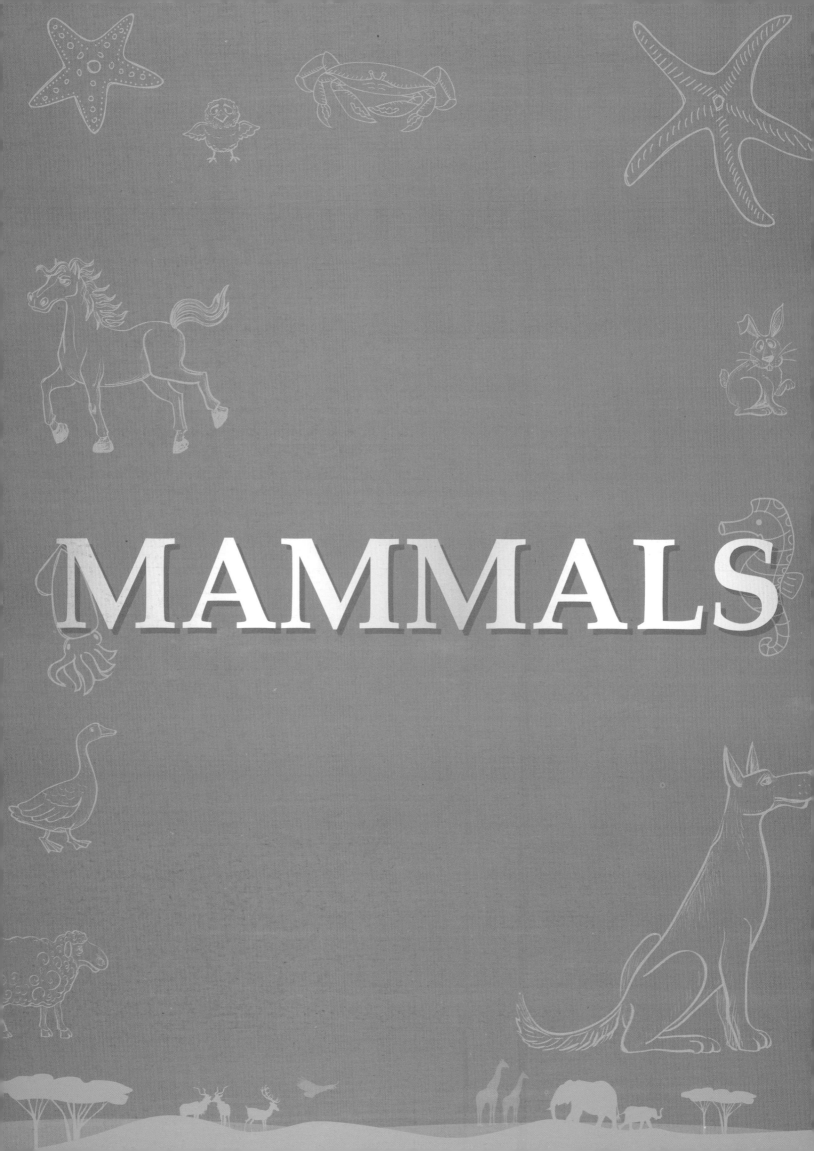

MAMMALS

THE WORLD OF MAMMALS

Mammals have lived on Earth for a long time! They are classified as species that give birth to their young (not by laying eggs), and whose females feed their babies with milk from their bodies. So, even human beings are classified as mammals.

The earliest known mammals were the tiny morganucodontids that lived 210 million years ago alongside the mighty dinosaurs. When a huge asteroid or comet struck Earth, the dinosaurs were wiped out and the mammals had a chance to grow and evolve.

Today, many diverse species of animals roam the Earth. Small mammals like the thumb-sized pygmy shrew and large mammals like the blue whale are a mark of mammalian diversity as are tall giraffes and flying bats. Read on to find out more about this vast group of animals.

▶ *Giraffes are the tallest mammals on our planet*

What Makes a Mammal?

Mammals are classified as 'Mammalia'. This class of animals have a few unique features that make them the highest order of beings residing on the planet. Besides giving birth to their young and feeding them milk from their own bodies, there are other features that determine whether an animal species is a mammal.

Hair

Hair refers to small thread-like projections that emerge from the outermost layer of the mammal's skin. It is also called the fur or animal coat. All mammals possess this trait, though they may have hair in varied appearances and at different stages of their lives.

Dolphins have small pits at the snout, where they had hair at the time of their birth. Dolphin calves in their mother's womb have these pits filled with hair, but after birth, the hairs fall off while swimming. Animals like elephants and rhinoceroses have sparse, bristly hair, while polar bears have a long, thick fur to keep warm in the cold Arctic. Human beings are among the mammals that have lesser hair.

Warm Blood

Mammals are warm-blooded animals. In other words, unlike amphibians or fish, they can maintain their body temperature, regardless of being out in the snow or sunlight. Their average body temperature varies between 36.7° C and 37.2° C. This ability of mammals to produce heat within their own bodies is called **endothermy**.

How do mammals maintain their body temperature? They might shiver. This action increases the heat that their bodies produce. To keep cool, they might pant or sweat, which leads to heat loss. Some mammals might hibernate. This reduces the heat in the body as other bodily functions slow down.

▲ Naked mole rats cannot control their body temperatures very well, so they like to live in tunnels to keep cool

▲ Polar bears need their fur to keep warm in freezing habitats

▶ A lioness with her cub; according to experts, there are only about 20,000 of these fierce cats left in the wild

Giving Birth

Majority of mammals (with the exceptions of the duck-billed platypus and echidna) do not lay eggs. The mother bears the young ones inside her body in an organ called the uterus until birth. Such organisms are called **viviparous**. Except for **marsupials**, who carry the young ones in a pouch, mammals give birth to a well-developed baby. The time the **foetus** spends in the womb of the mother is called the gestation period, which differs in all animals. An elephant carries its baby for almost 22 months, while the Virginia opossum carries its baby for only 12–13 days.

Mammalian Milk

Once the baby is born, it is fed milk produced by a special organ called mammary glands. This unique characteristic defines mammals. Non-functional glands are seen in males too, but it is the females which carry glands that can produce milk to feed the baby.

In primitive animals like the duck-billed platypus, the glands express milk directly onto the skin or fur, which is then lapped up by the baby. Mammary glands are modifications of sweat glands, the organ that produces sweat.

◀ Bats have extraordinary hearing abilities

More Mammalian Features

In all other forms of **vertebrates**, the jaw is attached to the skull via a set of bones. However, in mammals, early on during evolution, the jaw hinged itself directly to the skull, to create a set of ear bones; this helps this class of organisms hear better. Also, mammals have different types of teeth, such as the molars, premolars, canines, and incisors. These specialised teeth help them grind and chew their food. The biggest evolutionary development in mammals is their big brain, which helps them think and reason better.

🔦 Isn't It Amazing!

Humpback whales are very agile for their size. How does the huge animal manage to be so swift? That is because it has golf-ball sized bumps on its head and **pectoral fins**. They are **hair follicles** connected to sensitive nerves. Studies reveal it is these that help the whale in being swift. Also, the hair follicles are said to help the animal detect water currents and food.

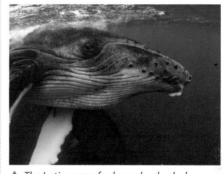

▲ The Latin name for humpback whales is 'Megaptera novaeangliae', meaning 'big wing of New England'

👤 In Real Life

Elephants can overheat easily because they do not have a large skin surface in comparison to their body size. These animals do not sweat like human beings; instead, they use their skin to keep cool. If the skin heats up on a hot day or after a long walk, the internal heat generated cannot be reduced. This is where their hair comes to the rescue. It helps the body stay cool!

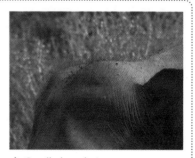

▲ Small, sharp hair seen on an elephant's head

A Blast from the Past

Though it might be hard to imagine, it took a long time for the different species of mammals to evolve into what we see today. If we want to read about the evolution of different mammals, we can do so because of the researchers and scientists who have unearthed fossils or remains of extinct mammals that existed long before the advent of human beings. Through the study of these fossils, scientists learned about the existence, behaviour, food habits, and extinction of ancient mammals.

Sabre-toothed Cats

If we were alive 42 million to 11,000 years ago, then we might have been able to spot sabre-toothed cats in the wild. Sadly, these mammals are extinct. They were said to live in North America and Europe as their fossils were found around these continents. There were different species of sabre-toothed cats and some of them prowled the wilds of South America too.

Sabre-toothed cats had short, bulky bodies and short tails when compared to modern lions. These vicious cats were known for their sabre-like teeth, which were very long and sharp. They were named after this feature.

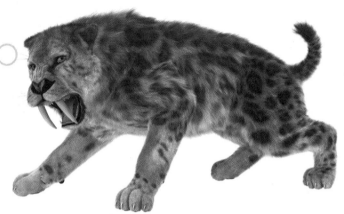

▲ It is misleading to call these animals sabre-toothed tigers as they are not closely related to modern tigers

▼ The Deinotherium is also called the 'Hoe-tusker'

Deinotherium

The name *Deinotherium* means 'terrible beast'. At a glance, this large ancient mammal resembles the modern elephant. But compare them closely and their differences become clear. The *Deinotherium* had a shorter trunk and downward-facing tusks. Scientists believe they were used to pull down trees or dig out roots from underground. It was also much larger than the modern elephant, nearly 13 feet tall. It lived in Europe, Asia, and Africa. The African species outlasted the other two. The mammal disappeared around 7 million years ago.

Isn't It Amazing!

Even though they are named for their famous teeth, it is believed that at least two species of the sabre-toothed cats had weak jaws and bites. These mammals did not chase their prey. Instead, they ambushed it with their packs. They bit the prey but primarily used their neck muscles and forelimbs to hold it down and weaken it. Research has revealed that modern lions might have stronger bites than these ancient beasts!

Glyptodont

Think of the armadillo. Now, picture a creature that is much larger in size and weighs nearly 2,000 kilograms. It is the glyptodont. Compared to that, the modern armadillo (a distant cousin) only weighs up to 54 kilograms!

The glyptodont originated about 20 million years ago. It had a powerful spiky tail that was shaped like a club. It had a tough **carapace**—the bony outer shell covered with scales. It lived in South America and is said to have disappeared at the end of the last Ice Age, about 10,000 years ago.

▶ *The extinction of glyptodonts coincided with the arrival of early humans in the Americas*

Entelodont

The extinct entelodonts and modern pigs share a long, extended family. They might even have been related to the modern hippopotamuses. Fossil evidence shows that the entelodonts originated about 40 million years ago and became extinct 16–19 million years ago. These ancient mammals roamed in Asia, Europe, and North America.

The animals were medium or large with the heaviest species found to be nearly 900 kilograms. Naturally, they were much heavier than the modern pigs. The entelodonts probably had an **omnivorous** diet.

◀ *The entelodont had a fierce temper and was extremely fast*

The Walking Whale

In 1992, a **paleontologist** named Hans Thewissen discovered the first fossil of a whale in Pakistan which was, at the time, about 49 million years old. This fossil was of an animal called *Ambulocetus natans*, which had four legs. They were of an older ancestor or relative of the whale called *Pakicetus*.

On examining the jaw and ear, Thewissen discovered that the fossil resembled the structure of a modern whale and had strong hind limbs. He believed that the whale's ancestors began to evolve into their aquatic lifestyle nearly 50 million years ago.

In Real Life

Along with the sabre-toothed cat, the woolly mammoths make the movie *Ice Age* interesting. In reality, they were as big as African elephants but had small ears, probably to keep out the cold of the Ice Age. They had very long tusks and were herbivores. They disappeared when the climate turned warmer.

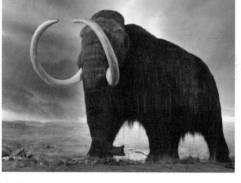

▲ *As the name suggests, the woolly mammoth's body was covered with woolly hair to keep warm*

Incredible Individuals

Hans Thewissen is a Dutch paleontologist and a researcher in the field of anatomy. He focuses on the study of whale fossils to understand how they evolved from land animals. He is also involved in the conservation of beluga whales and does fieldwork in Asia, Alaska, and the neighbouring regions.

Mammalian Orders

Modern mammals are a diverse set. They may share common features, but they are different from each other. This could be due to environmental adaptations. The small shrew, the large elephant, the carnivorous tiger, and the intelligent ape are all mammals.

Classification of Mammals

Scientists have classified mammals into several groups. Each group consists of animals bearing characteristics that are largely similar to each other. This classification, based on newer research, is subject to change.

01

Monotremes (order Monotremata)

Identifier: Egg-laying mammals

Characteristics: These mammals lay eggs instead of giving birth to young ones.

Example: Duck-billed platypus

02

Marsupials (infraclass Marsupialia)

Identifier: Pouched animals

Characteristics: These mammals give birth to their young in the abdominal pouch. Their gestation period is short, and the young one is born as an immature foetus that lives in the pouch until it develops fully.

Example: Kangaroo

03

Even-toed Ungulates (order Cetartiodactyla)

Identifier: Even-toed mammals

Characteristics: The group includes land-dwelling even-toed ungulates like camels, deers, cattle, hippopotamuses. Marine mammals like whales and dolphins also belong to this group.

Example: Deer

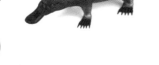

04

Cetaceans (infraorder Cetacea)

Identifier: Aquatic mammals

Characteristics: These mammals are quite unique as they are aquatic, have dorsal fins, flippers in the front, and **blubber** and **blowholes**. They are closely related to hippopotami.

Examples: Dolphin

05 Carnivores (order Carnivora)

Identifier: Flesh-eaters

Characteristics: Carnivorous mammals have large canine teeth and blade-like molars. Most such mammals live on land. Some carnivores are domesticated.

Example: Fox, cat, walrus

06 Pinnipeds (suborder Pinnipedia)

Identifier: Fin-footed

Characteristics: A subgroup of carnivores called 'pinnipeds' live in the water. Their feet have evolved into flippers for swimming.

Example: Seal

07

Bats (order Chiroptera)

Identifier: Flying mammals

Characteristics: Bats are the only mammals who are capable of true flight. Membranes stretch between the fingers of their hands. They use echolocation (sonar echoes) to navigate.

Example: Vampire Bat

08 Lagomorphs (order Lagomorpha)

Identifier: Hare-shaped
Characteristics: These mammals have long ears, short tails, and hind legs adapted to bouncing movements.
Example: Rabbit

09 Odd-toed Ungulates (order Perissodactyla)

Identifier: Odd-toed and hoofed
Characteristics: They are herbivores with an odd number of toes. They consume food by grazing or **browsing**.
Example: Horse

10 Xenarthrans (Superorder Xenarthra)

Identifier: Toothless mammals
Characteristics: Different species have underdeveloped or no molar teeth. They do not have incisors. They dig the ground and eat insects. Their spines are rigid.
Example: Armadillo

11 Colugo (order Dermoptera)

Identifier: Gliding mammals
Characteristics: Dermoptera are also called flying lemurs or colugos. These mammals glide from tree to tree.
Example: Ring-tailed lemur

12 Primates (order Primates)

Identifier: Big-brained
Characteristics: They have large brains, good vision, and dexterous hands. Many even have **opposable thumbs**.
Example: Chimpanzee

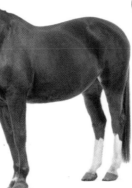

13 Aardvarks (order Tubulidentata)

Identifier: Tubular teeth
Characteristics: They are nocturnal and termite-eating mammals.
Example: Aardvark

14 Rodents (order Rodentia)

Identifier: Largest order of mammals
Characteristics: They are small herbivores with sharp incisors. There are 1,500 living species of rodents.
Example: Squirrel

15 Insectivores (order Eulipotyphla)

Identifier: Insect-eaters
Characteristics: They eat insects and have snouts. They have a good sense of smell and live in burrows or trees.
Example: Hedgehog

16 Pangolins (order Pholidata)

Identifier: Scaly mammals
Characteristics: There are only eight pangolin species alive today. They are covered with scales, and eat ants and termites.
Example: Tree hyrax

17 Hyraxes (order Hyracoidea)

Identifier: Diurnal or nocturnal
Characteristics: These animals are small hooved and have a rodent-like appearance. They are herbivores. While other hooved animals use their incisors to crop their food, the rock hyraxes use their molars.
Example: Tree hyrax

18 Sirenians (order Sirenia)

Identifier: Aquatic herbivores
Characteristics: TThey live in the waters of tropical and sub-tropical regions. They have front flippers and no hind limbs. These slow mammals eat underwater plants. There are five surviving species of this order.
Example: Manatee

19 Elephants (order Proboscidea)

Identifier: Trunk-nosed mammals
Characteristics: All mammals belonging to this order have trunks. They grab food and drink water using their trunks. They are large herbivorous mammals that graze and browse food.

Example: African elephant

The Carnivore at the Top

Mammalian predators hunt and eat flesh. For this purpose, they need sharp teeth to tear down the meat. Such animals are called carnivores. Polar bears, lions, killer whales, tigers, and wolves are predators. Few mammals such as coyotes are scavengers as well, which means they eat the meat of animals hunted by others. Polar bears are the world's largest terrestrial carnivores.

◀ *Polar bears have no fear of other animals as they do not have any natural predators*

◀ *Less than 2 per cent of polar bear hunts are successful*

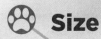 Habitat

Polar bears are found in countries surrounding the Arctic Circle near the North Pole. They live in Greenland, Canada, Russia, and Norway. Polar bears are not found in Antarctica. Instead, they roam around the vast empty ice fields of the Arctic in search of food.

Size

Polar bears have long necks, short heads, and short tails which are about 7–13 cm long. They are hefty and strong animals who are at the top of the food chain in their habitat.

⊛ Incredible Individuals

Imagine that your friends had never heard of the polar bear. How would you describe it to them? The first recorded sighting of a polar bear was made by William Burrough (1537–1598), who was a navigator from Europe. He, along with the members on his ship *Serchthrift*, witnessed a hunting party chase a polar bear. Another explorer, John Davis (1550–1605), described them as a 'monstrous bigness'. Nearly two centuries later, a man named Constantine John Phipps (1744–1792) described the bears in detail and gave them their scientific name, *Ursus maritimus,* (which translates to sea bear), in his 1774 account *A Voyage Towards the North Pole*.

🐾 Trapping Warmth

Polar bears live in the freezing Arctic, so they need to keep themselves warm. They have thick fur in the form of long, hollow hair for insulation. Also, their bodies are covered with a thick layer of fat called blubber that protects them from the harsh winters. While their fur is white, their skin is black and absorbs heat.

🐾 Keen Smell

Polar bears have a keen sense of smell. They use it to hunt seals, their favourite prey. It is said that polar bears can smell as far as 9 kilometres away. Once they find a seal's breathing hole, that it creates to come out of the water and breathe, they wait patiently for hours for the seal to emerge so that they can attack it.

🐾 Swimming Champions

In one hour, polar bears can swim up to 10 km. Unlike all other four-legged animals, they only use their front limbs to swim. They can swim continuously for hours and have even been known to swim hundreds of kilometres without stopping. But these bears are unsuccessful when it comes to hunting in the open waters. That is why they need to look for seals' breathing holes. When they are swimming under water, they close their nostrils and the blubber keeps them warm.

🐾 Eating Habits

Polar bears eat seals but they also eat small mammals, birds, bird eggs, and even plants. This is because they are omnivores.

▲ Polar bears are also called sea bears for their swimming prowess

🐾 Giving Birth

Polar bears have a long gestation period that lasts around 195–265 days. Female polar bears give birth to young ones in the winter. After they mate, female polar bears try to gain at least 200 kg in weight as that is necessary for them to successfully give birth. They birth the young ones in snow dens which protect the mother and cub from the cold winters.

Female bears dig the dens; they are long tunnels with a narrow entrance. A female polar bear will give birth once in three years. They mostly have twins, while single cubs and triplets are less common. Cubs barely weigh around 680 grams when born. They are weak and have their eyes closed. The mother nurses them with its four mammary glands. Once winter is over, the bear family surfaces from the den. Cubs stay with their mothers for about two years to learn how to become independent.

🐾 Not So Good News

Polar bears move from one ice floe (floating ice sheet) to another when they hunt for seals. With rapid climatic changes taking place, often there is not much ice in the Arctic during summers. With so much ice melting, the bears (although they are good swimmers) must swim long distances between floes. Thus, exhausted polar bears drown before reaching their destination. Polar bears are in the International Union for Conservation of Nature (IUCN) list of vulnerable animals and their biggest enemy is climate change and human beings who hunt them.

The Killer Whale

Though they live in the water, the killer whales, or orcas, are some of the most fierce and predatory animals on the Earth. With a large, powerful build that supports a top speed of 56 kmph, and a smart, cunning mind, the killer whale is very well named.

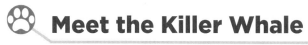 Meet the Killer Whale

Killer whales are also called orcas. Do not be confused by the name though, because they are technically dolphins. These giant carnivores are around 20–26 feet in size and 6,000–10,000 kilograms in weight. They are so large and fierce that they do not have a natural predator. The biggest threat to their existence is human beings.

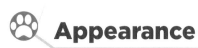 Appearance

Imagine that you have lost a tooth, but it does not grow back again. That is what happens to killer whales. They only have one set of teeth which are large and interlocking. Killer whales have 40–56 teeth; each is about 7.6 centimetres long. They are sharp and can tear apart the prey easily.

The black and white skin of killer whales is constantly renewed. Therefore, they have very smooth skin that helps them swim fast. They have 7.6-10 centimetre thick layer of blubber beneath their skin.

Diet

Killer whales do not chew their food, they swallow it whole. They eat sea lions, small seals, penguins, walruses, squids, sharks, and fish. Orcas eat about 230 kilograms of food daily.

▲ *Orcas stick to family groups called 'pods'*

Predatory Nature

Killer whales do not have the playful nature that their cousins—the dolphins—are famous for. They might be smart and social like dolphins, but they are also dangerous—one of the top predators of the sea. They live in large pods or family groups. All members of the pod participate in hunting. They hunt using strategies very similar to wolves, such as encircling the prey before moving in for the kill.

Killer whales have black backs, but their stomachs are white. So, a seal sitting on an ice floe might not see the whale, because the black blends well with the water.

They sneak up on and bump off the seal from the floe, into the water, to catch it. Similarly, a fish might not see the white underside as it blends with the light streaming down in the sea from the surface.

◀ *Killer whales also eat krill to maintain their body weight*

The Intelligent Dolphins

Dolphins are warm-blooded mammals and not fish, despite living under water. They belong to the family of cetaceans—a group that also includes porpoises, orcas, and whales. Most dolphins have a small build of around 6.2-8.2 feet. They have streamlined bodies, a pointed snout, and sharp teeth.

Behaviour

Dolphins are remarkably intelligent and playful marine mammals. They are predominantly found in the shallow waters of tropical or temperate regions. Just like bats, they use echolocation to navigate the waters and hunt for fish, squids, and crustaceans. To conserve energy, dolphins bow-ride and swim alongside ships. They are known for their grace and playfulness.

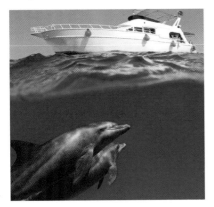

▲ *Dolphins bow-riding with a boat*

A Dolphin at Rest

Unlike human beings, who can breathe subconsciously, dolphins have to consciously take air into their lungs. They do not have gills, like fish. Instead, they breathe through a blowhole, which is a nostril located on top of their heads. When dolphins sleep, one part of their brain switches off, while the other remains alert to keep breathing. They switch sides in approximately two hours and the other part of the brain wakes up, watching for predators and signalling when to come up for fresh air. This is called catnapping. Individual dolphins enter into a deeper form of sleep, usually in the night, called logging. This name comes from the fact that a dolphin looks like a log floating in the water while it is in deep sleep.

Smiling Dolphins

Bottlenose dolphins are amongst the most popular dolphin species and commonly perform at oceanariums because of their great communication abilities. If you look at the dolphin's face shown here, it looks like it is always smiling because of the curvature of its mouth. Every dolphin has a unique whistling sound. Bottlenose dolphins can remember and recognise the sound of each dolphin, even after they are separated for 10 to 20 years.

Parenting

Female dolphins sleep on the move so that they can take care of the young by towing them along in their slipstream. This is called echelon swimming. Baby dolphins need a lot of rest and sleep and will drown if their mother does not carry them to the surface. While looking after newborns, the mothers cannot sleep for weeks at a time as baby dolphins are not born with enough blubber to keep them afloat. They stay with their mothers till they are eight years old. Dolphins also travel in pairs and sleep while slowly swimming with each other.

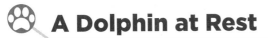

▲ *The 'smiling' bottlenose dolphin*

◀ *Dolphins can live in groups of as few as five and as many as hundreds. They are social learners*

Predators of the Night

Bats are commonly mistaken for birds because they can fly, but they are mammals. They emerge at night and sleep during the day. These flying mammals come in varied sizes; the tiniest one being the bumblebee bat, with a wing span of up to 17 centimetres. Many species of bats live on fruits, while vampire bats drink the blood of other animals.

▶ *Some bats can achieve flight speeds of up to 160 kmph*

Vampire Bats

Vampire bats rest in caves, hollows of trees, and abandoned buildings. They live in Mexico, Central America, and South America. These mammals live in groups ranging from 100 to 1,000.

Vampire bats have a lifespan of about 12 years. They are small, with a length of 7 or 9 centimetres and a weight of about 15–45 grams.

A Bloody Affair

Unlike the mythical creatures they are named after, vampire bats do not suck blood. They make a small cut on their prey with their teeth and drink the blood that flows out. These bats are so agile that at times they can drink blood from an animal or bird for 30 minutes before waking them up. The prey is not harmed, but might get infections.

▲ *Most bats hang upside down while resting*

Vampire bats usually drink blood from pigs, cows, horses and birds. These bats have important adaptations which help them in feeding. They have a heat sensor on their nose which helps them find warm blood flowing through the victim. While feeding, their saliva prevents blood from clotting. The young vampire bats do not drink blood but feed on their mother's milk instead for almost three months after birth. They cling to the mother even while she is in flight.

Incredible Individuals

An Italian scientist named Lazzaro Spallanzani (1729–1799) discovered that bats were able to navigate through hurdles and find their prey even if they were blinded. He made several discoveries about how the bodies of bats function and how they reproduce.

Echolocation

Bats have very small eyes and extremely sensitive sight. They cannot see colours like human beings, but they can see in the dark. As they hunt at night, vampire bats also use **echolocation**. It means that bats send sound waves with their mouth or nose. These bounce off on surfaces like the walls of a cave and echo back to the bat. The signal is enough for it to identify a prey (its size or location) and any hurdles.

The Prowling Tiger

There are many species of tigers, with the Bengal tigers being one of the most famous ones. They can be easily spotted because of their bright orange-reddish coats with unique dark stripes. They are found in very diverse habitats such as tropical forests, grasslands, swamps, rocky terrains, and even colder regions like Siberia.

🐾 Behaviour

Tigers are the biggest cats in the big cat family that includes leopards, lions, and cheetahs. They have three-foot long tails which allow them to maintain balance. On average, they weigh between 100 to 350 kilograms, stand around 3 feet tall and have sharp claws. The mammals use their claws to swiftly kill their prey.

Tigers are solitary hunters. Their agility makes them very dangerous. They usually prey on deer, antelopes, pigs, water buffaloes, and even horses. They are mostly nocturnal mammals that hunt every 4–7 days and can eat up to 10 kilograms of meat in one sitting. Tigers always know when they are in another tiger's territory because they mark their territories with their urine or by scratching the nearby trees.

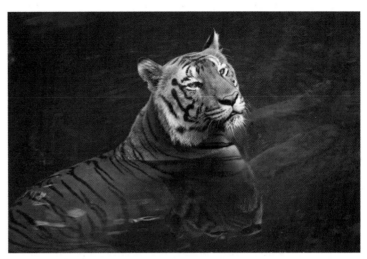

▲ *Tigers are great swimmers. The Bengal tiger cools off by taking a quick swim and splashes around in the water*

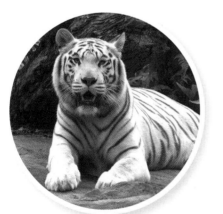

▶ *White or bleached tigers are seen in India. They are quite rare. They are not a separate species from Bengal tigers, but just have a different pigmentation*

🐾 A Tiger's Roar

In the early 1900s, there were over 100,000 tigers roaming around in their territories, but today their numbers have reduced greatly. Tigers are now considered to be an endangered species. They have dwindled in population primarily because of poaching, hunting, and loss of habitat. Today, not more than 4,000 tigers exist in the world.

▼ *Tigers are often hunted for their skin and teeth*

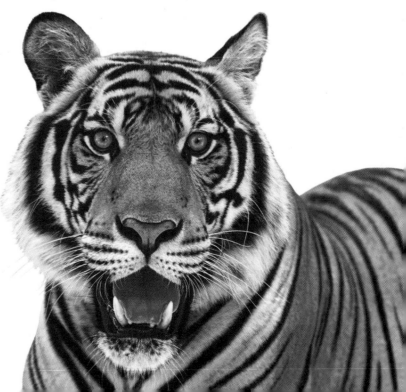

Species	Status
Bengal tiger	Less than 2,000
Indochinese tiger	Around 350
Siberian/Amur tiger	Around 500
Sumatran tiger	Less than 400
Malayan tiger	Less than 200
South Chinese tiger	Extinct in the wild; bred in captivation
Caspian tiger	Extinct
Javan tiger	Extinct
Bali tiger	Extinct

The Agile Fox

Foxes do not hunt in packs, unlike their wolf cousins. Instead, they hunt extra prey and bury it away for later. This behaviour has probably contributed to their 'sly' reputation. The fox is popularly mentioned in legends where it is portrayed primarily as cunning or intelligent. The male fox is called reynard and the female fox, vixen. Foxes belong to the larger canine family called Canidae, of which dogs are also a part.

🐾 Special Features

Though they are related to dogs, foxes have cat-like retractable claws and vertical pupils. They have a slender frame, thin legs, a pointed nose, and a bushy tail. Grey foxes are the only canines that can climb trees to escape attackers.

Foxes easily adapt to numerous kinds of habitats and exist in every continent except Antarctica. They use their nocturnal abilities to hunt mice, birds, frogs, insects, fruits, and seeds, as they are omnivores.

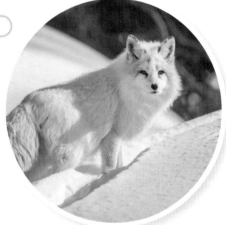

▶ *The artic or polar fox uses its white fur to camouflage itself in the snow against predators*

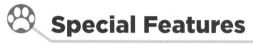

▼ *Red foxes can be very agile, jumping to even 7 feet to cross a fence*

🐾 The Red Fox

There are 37 types of foxes, but the red fox is the most common. Its natural habitat can range from arid deserts to the Arctic tundra. They are spotted in Australia and Central America. Red foxes are small creatures, generally about 90–105 centimetres long, of which 35-40 cm is the tail and weigh just 5–7 kilograms. This is the same weight as that of a one-year-old baby.

Red foxes have adapted so well to the human environment that they are now considered pets in Australia. They can be found in woods, farmlands, and many large suburbs.

🐾 What Does the Fox Say?

Foxes seem to have a lot to talk about. They are extremely vocal animals, and have at least 28 different types of calls, 8 of which are only used by their cubs.

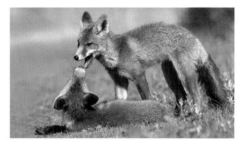

Contact call: It is made by two foxes as they approach each other. It sounds similar to a dog's bark, but is of a higher pitch, like an owl's hoot. Once the foxes make physical contact, they have a greeting call that sounds like a chicken's clucking.

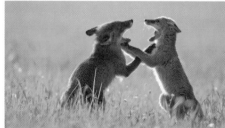

Interaction call: These sounds vary based on social status and how aggressive the fox is. A submissive fox will let out a high-pitched whine when facing an aggressive fox. They also make a clicking sound called gekkering when they are feeling playful or aggressive.

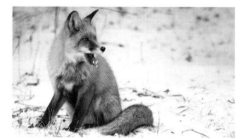

Alarm call: These are made by parents to warn each other about oncoming danger. It sounds like a sharp 'waaaah'. The vixen's scream is another terrifying and loud sound made in anguish.

The Galloping Horse

Horses belong to the Equidae family. They comprise a singular species called *Equus caballus*. There are many different breeds within this species. Horses are a common sight because human beings have domesticated them and used them as means of transportation for centuries. A male horse is called a stallion and a female horse is called a mare. Young horses are known as foals.

Features

Horses are animals of speed. They have long, firm legs with hooves they use to gallop. Their compact bodies are supported by the tips of their toes, allowing their limbs to extend forward and gain speed. They have large and complex brains in their well-rounded skulls. This allows for great muscle coordination.

Horses weigh between 350–1,000 kilograms. As they are herbivores, they have a set of sharp, high-crowned teeth that they use to graze and grind grass. Horses also have long digestive tracts to digest cellulose from vegetation. Their diet consists of hay, grain and water. They need sugar and lots of salt, which they can get from vegetables and fruits.

Behaviour

Horses have developed sensory systems for good memory, accurate judgement and strong instincts. They are social herd animals. Their intrinsic nature is to actively seek out a mutually beneficial relationship. They do not fare well in isolation. Human beings have exploited this trait and domesticated them for centuries. Horses scare easily and only get aggressive when they are mistreated or cannot flee.

How Do Horses Sleep?

Human beings tend to sleep at a stretch for eight hours. Horses do not do this. They rest for short periods, many times a day. Their sleeping patterns change depending upon their age and the weather. They cannot sleep well in the cold. Till the age of three months, young foals spend half their day sleeping by lying down. As they grow older, they sleep standing up. For adult horses, lying down can be more challenging than standing, so they only lie down for a short time.

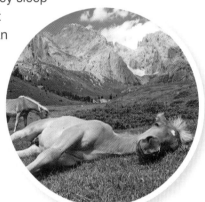

▶ *Horses need about three hours of sleep each day*

▼ *Horses have strong instincts that allow them to sense distant danger. They can even sense the emotional temperament of their riders*

In Real Life

Horses have played a very important role in human civilisation for centuries now. They were used by kings and soldiers in combat and warfare. They routinely feature in art as steady companions for human beings. For centuries, human beings have been heavily reliant on these animals for transportation. Literature often depicts horses as the vehicle of choice for noble heroes and the gods. Today, riding horses has become a recreational sport. Horses are also at the centre of various sports from polo to horse racing, and were used for jousting in the medieval era. They were also used to make glue as they, among other animals, contain a lot of collagen, a protein found in connective tissue, hide, and bone. It is evident that horses and humans go a long way back.

The Graceful Deer

Reindeers have often been associated with Christmas tales, and are well-known all over the world. They belong to the deer family. Except for Australia and Antarctica, deers are native to every continent. They are noted for having two large and two small hooves on each foot. Male deers have strong antlers in most species, while only female reindeers have antlers. They shed and regrow these antlers every year. Deers also have scent glands on their legs but do not have rectal or vulval glands; they do not have a gall bladder either.

Diet

Since deer have very complex digestive organs, they are very specialised herbivores. They feed on grasses, fruits, aquatic plants, and herbs that contain protein and are easily digestible. Due to this limitation, they cannot sustain themselves in deserts, dry grasslands, or leached faunas. Deer have learnt to identify disturbed ecosystems and use it to their advantage. If there has been a flood, a wildfire, or an avalanche, they exploit the nutrient-rich landscape the disaster leaves in its wake.

Behaviour

Deer belonging to different sets of fauna differ in their survival tactics. Those who belong to forests can easily hide in the thick of the forest. Those who belong to a flat terrain tend to be specialised runners and can bolt at the sign of danger. Deer who live on rocky terrains tend to be specialised jumpers and can explore high altitudes that are inaccessible to their predators.

▼ Deer are seen as gentle animals, often skittish and nervous around predators. If they sense danger, they take off running

Reindeers

Also referred to as caribou, reindeer live in the far northern regions of North America, Europe, and Asia. They are found in the Arctic tundra and nearby forests. They are the most domesticated species of deer, often used as pets and to pull sleighs in the snow. The antlers of male reindeer can grow up to 4.3 feet, making them look magnificent. They are exceptional swimmers and their coats are well-insulated. Their cloven hoofs are deep and thus, they are able to walk on soft ground and snow.

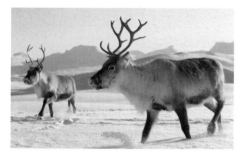

▲ Reindeer's noses are specially designed to warm the air before it reaches their lungs

💡 Isn't It Amazing!

During harsh winters, reindeers survive on a particular lichen due to a lack of vegetation. They supplement this by recycling urea, which is normally a waste product. They do it within their digestive system by using up all the nitrogen present in the urea. Males shed their antlers during such periods, but females keep them throughout winter to defend themselves from other deer trying to share their food.

The Unique Rodents

Rodents are the largest group of mammals, having over 2,050 living species. They have 27 separate families such as porcupines, mice, beavers, and squirrels, among others. They are characterised by their rootless incisor teeth which are coated with thick enamel. They eat their food by gnawing, and thus their teeth have very chiselled edges. Rodents have to keep gnawing as their incisor teeth never stop growing.

Size

Rodents are small creatures. The largest living one is the capybara, which weighs around 35-66 kilograms on average. Most rodents do not live longer than a year, but some of the larger ones, like beavers, live almost till they are 20 years of age. As a result of their short lifespans, they have very fast reproductive cycles and achieve sexual maturity very quickly.

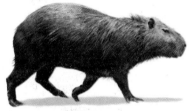

▲ *Capybaras are extremely friendly; they interact with about every other animal*

Diet

The dietary behaviour of rodents changes according to the species. Their preferences can be set apart using various classifications such as diet patterns, and hunting or gathering styles. Rodents may be herbivorous or omnivorous. They have species which might live an adaptable lifestyle of being hunters as the opportunity presents itself, or being specialists e.g. the grasshopper mouse hunts arthropods, while some rodents hunt vertebrates.

Beavers

Beavers are the second-largest rodents with bodies extending up to 120 cm. They are primarily nocturnal and amphibious creatures that live in rivers, streams, marshes, and ponds. They have short legs and a stout body with a small, broad, and blunt head. As herbivores, their diet consists mostly of bark, leaves, twigs, roots, and aquatic plants.

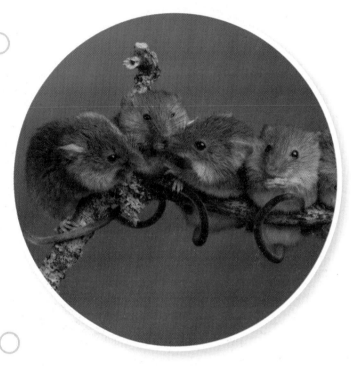

▲ *Mice live close to their food source and build colonies near human homes. Their rapid growth in population can prove to be quite tiresome for human beings*

Mice

A mouse is a small nocturnal mammal with a pointed snout, small rounded ears, and an almost hairless tail which can grow as long as its body. Mice have poor eyesight but a keen sense of smell and hearing. There are more than 30 known species of these rodents. The house mouse is a popular pet and other mouse species seen in and around the house are the field mouse, the American white-footed mouse, and the deer mouse. They are widely hunted by cats, wild dogs, foxes, birds of prey, and snakes. In their natural habitat mice are herbivores that eat all kinds of fruit and grains from plants. Using their whiskers to sense changes in temperature, mice build winding burrows with many escape routes.

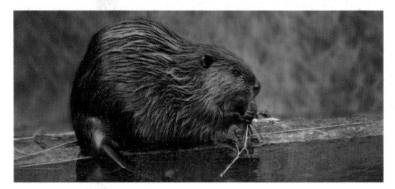

◀ *Beavers can use their incisors to block the water from entering their mouth as they cut branches growing under the water's surface*

The Herbivorous Hippo

A hippopotamus looks aggressive and strong, so it is often thought to be a carnivore, but it is herbivorous. Herbivores eat grass and leaves. Mammals like giraffes, cows, elephants, sheep, and goats are some more examples of herbivores. These animals have flat and wide molar teeth to grind the grasses and leaves, unlike predators who need sharp canine teeth to cut and bite into flesh.

Aggressive Hippos

Hippopotamuses look docile, slow, and sluggish, but they can get aggressive when they feel threatened. On land, they can run at the speed of 15 kmph and even reach a speed of 30 kmph for short distances. There have been incidents when they have killed buffaloes, impalas, as well as human beings. Even a ferocious predator like a lion cannot take on a hippo on its own and needs to hunt it in pairs.

Habitat

Hippopotamuses look for food on land, but water is essential to their habitats. In fact, their name translates to 'river horse'. Once, they were found all over Africa, but are now confined to some parts of East and West Africa. Due to habitat loss and hunting, they are now listed as a vulnerable species.

Size

Hippopotamuses have barrel-shaped bodies, short legs and tails, and large heads. Their skin can be greyish or brownish, with blotches of faded pink on the underside. They can weigh as much as around 3,000 kilograms, making them the second-largest terrestrial animal living in the world.

Cooling Effect

Hippopotamuses stay in places with hot climates. To cool themselves off, they spend their days in rivers and lakes. Interestingly, they produce a natural substance that acts like suntan lotion when they sweat. It is an oily red liquid which protects their skin from the Sun and prevents drying.

Herds

Hippopotamuses live in groups of ten or twenty. The herd has a dominant male who is protective of the group. The others in the herd are the females, young ones, and non-breeding males. To keep other males away, male hippopotamuses open their mouth wide to display their long, razor-sharp canines. They are also known to make loud noises and splash aggressively in water.

Female hippos, also known as cows, give birth to a single calf every two years. They stick to their herd as it offers protection against predators such as crocodiles and lions.

The hippopotamus is considered to be the most dangerous animal in Africa

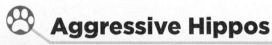

The Strong Elephant

Elephants are the largest terrestrial animals on Earth. They are known for their distinctively long noses or trunks, large; floppy ears; and wide, thick legs. The two major types of elephants, the Asian elephant and the African elephant inhabit separate continents.

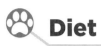

Diet

Their diet consists of grasses, roots, fruits, and bark. They use their tusks to pull the bark from trees and dig roots out of the ground. These giants spend a majority of their day feeding. An adult can eat 136 kg of food in a day.

Reproduction

Male elephants are referred to as 'bulls' and females as 'cows'. Post copulation, the cow's period of gestation is around 22 months. When the baby elephant is finally delivered, it can weigh around 91 kilograms and stand 3 feet tall. A baby elephant is called a 'calf'. The calf gains 1 kilogram every day up until it is one year old. By the time they are two years old, calves are ready to be weaned. Male calves leave, while females stay with the herd.

▼ African elephants are the largest land animals in the world

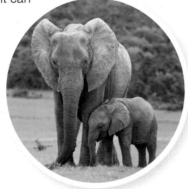

▲ Young elephants have no survival instinct; they rely on their mothers completely

Asian Elephant	African Elephant
Asian elephants grow up to 6.5-11.5 feet from shoulder to toe and weigh 2,500–5,500 kilograms.	African elephants can grow 8.2–13 feet from shoulder to toe and weigh 4,000-7,000 kilograms.
They live in Nepal, India, and Southeast Asia in scrub forests and rainforests.	These elephants inhabit sub-Saharan Africa, the rain forests of Central and West Africa, and the Sahel desert in Mali.
These elephants have smaller, round ears.	They have much larger ears shaped a bit like the continent of Africa.
Asian elephants have twin-domed heads, which means there is a divot line running up the head.	African elephants have rounded heads.

Behaviour

A group of elephants is called a herd. It is led by a matriarch, which is the oldest female. The matriarch is known to train the calves on how to behave amongst the community, which is a strong, close-knit family. Females, as well as young and old elephants stick together in a herd. Adult males tend to wander on their own.

Elephants display many strong emotions and instincts like empathy, mischief, and mourning. They sometimes hug by wrapping their trunks together in displays of greeting and affection or even respect, as taught by the matriarch. Elephants also use their distinctive trunks to help lift or nudge an elephant calf over an obstacle or to pull them out from a mud pit.

◄ Asian elephant

All About Marsupials

Similar to other mammals, marsupials have hair and mammary glands. Over 250 species of marsupials exist. They are characterised by the continued development and maternal dependency of their newborns.

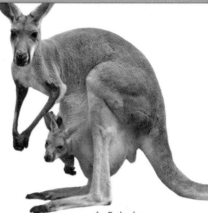

▲ *Baby kangaroos are known as joeys*

Young Marsupials

The young are very vulnerable at the time of their birth and are heavily reliant on the mother's milk. They fasten their mouth firmly on the mother's swollen up teats, and continue to develop for months in her marsupium. The marsupium or the pouch is a flap of skin that covers the mother's lower abdomen and teats. After a few months of warmth and shelter in the mother's pouch, the baby is gradually weaned off.

The Anteater

If you see an anteater, you will wonder how this toothless, strange-looking animal functions. They have a very long, worm-like tongue that helps them gulp down termites and ants easily. They have a tube-like snout and powerful, big claws that can tear down strong anthills. Their eyes and ears are small and rounded and they have very poor eyesight and hearing. Their brain is round and small too. But it is interesting how the anteaters' sense of smell is considered to be 40 times stronger than that of human beings! They live in tropical grasslands and forests in Central and South America. Anteaters easily eat a few thousand ants in one sitting and then abandon the nest. The biggest species are over 40 kilograms.

▲ *The biggest species of anteaters is the giant anteater*

Isn't It Amazing!

The modern kangaroo is a herbivore. Can you imagine a kangaroo that eats flesh? There was an extinct marsupial called *Ekaltadeta* closely related to the cute, jumpy kangaroos of today. They are also known as the killer kangaroo. As big as the modern dog, these killer kangaroos had large teeth and held down their prey with their front legs.

Koala

Koalas, also referred to as koala bears, are not bears, but are marsupials. They live in Australia on eucalyptus trees. They can eat more than a pound of leaves in a day. Mind you, they are fussy eaters and only choose the best leaves. They do not drink much water as they get all the water they need from the leaves they eat. The animals sleep more than 18 hours a day. A koala baby, when born is called the joey, and is blind and earless.

Kangaroos

Kangaroos are large animals that hop from place to place, at speeds as high as 56 kmph. They travel far and wide in search of food and water. These mammals have a pouch in which they carry their joey and belong to the *Macropodidae* family of marsupials that includes the happy quokkas and wallaroos.

▲ *Koalas eat up to 1 kg of eucalyptus leaves every day*

The Playful Seal

Seals belong to a species of web-footed aquatic mammals found in frigid water bodies. They have been known to live for more than 30 years. Some seals even make caves of snow to live in, while others never leave the ice pack and poke breathing holes in the ice. They are elegant and brisk swimmers owing to their structure, which has a rounded middle that tapers toward the ends.

Classification

There are two types of seals classified according to whether they have ears or are earless: True seals and eared seals. True seals are earless, while the eared seals comprise the sea lions and fur seals who have ears. Seals are carnivores, eating mainly fish, though some also consume squid, other molluscs, and crustaceans.

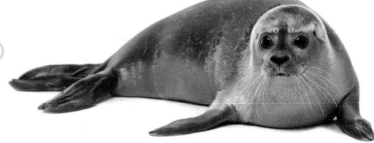
▲ A seal's whiskers help in detecting prey in dark, murky waters

True seals are more streamlined than fur seals and sea lions, and can therefore swim more effectively over long distances. However, because they cannot turn their hind flippers downwards, they are very clumsy on land, having to wriggle with their front flippers and abdominal muscles. This method of locomotion is called galumphing.

Migration of Elephant Seals

There are two types of elephant seals; the northern and the southern. The southern ones live in Antarctica, while the northern ones are seen on rocky beaches of northern oceans. It is there that they **moult**, sleep, mate, and give birth to young ones. However, the beaches are not their permanent abodes, in fact they spend more time in the ocean. These seals are known to migrate. They go migrating into the northern Pacific Ocean in the hunt for food, which gives them enough energy reserves for land-based activities. Interestingly, the male and female elephant seals like to migrate separately. Males travel nearly 21,000 kilometres in one year, while females travel almost 18,000 kilometres. Males fast for four months while they are on land and females fast for two months. All these different schedules make for a complicated migration season!

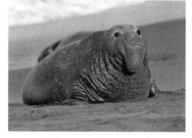
▲ Elephant seals can hold their breath for over 100 minutes

Social Beings

Seals are social animals that gather in large groups on beaches or masses of ice for the purpose of breeding. Male seals are called 'bulls', females are known as 'cows', and the baby seals are called 'pups'. Usually, seals form pairs during the period of procreation but some exceptions exist amongst the species. The gestation period lasts about 11 months. They give birth in dugouts of snow or on the open ice. The mother is known to stay out of water and not feed while she nurses the pup. The offspring acquire weight rapidly and stay on land till their waterproof fur grows.

On the Decline

Seals are hunted by killer whales, polar bears, leopard seals, large sharks, and human beings. Their species have seen a severe and rapid decrease in numbers in recent years. Many factors, including overfishing of other species, shooting by fishermen, and pollution have contributed to the decline.

◀ Cape fur seals are often seen nibbling on rocks

The Intelligent Primates

Scientists are known to have studied the teeth of primates to make findings about them. Around 57 million years ago, there lived a mammal which was probably the first true primate to have ever lived. It was a small animal named *'Altiatlasius'*. Its fossil was discovered in Morocco. Scientists feel it could be an important link in the evolution of primates.

What are Primates?

▶ *Some trainers have managed to train chimpanzees to perform sign language as part of an experiment*

A primate is mammalian group which includes monkeys, lemurs, tarsiers, apes, and human beings. Primates have big brains and are intelligent animals. Their eyes look straight ahead from their face.

Each of their hands has five fingers and each hind limb or foot has five toes. Primates are dexterous, meaning they can use their hands skilfully. Some ape species and human beings even have opposable thumbs.

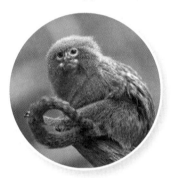

World's Smallest Monkey

It is the pygmy marmoset. It is so small that it can fit in the human palm and is found mainly in Brazil, Peru, and Colombia. These monkeys can leap up to 5 metres and can turn their heads backwards.

These adaptations help the pygmy marmoset scan the surroundings for predators. An interesting feature of this monkey is that while it is in conversation with others of its kind, it waits for its turn to speak.

▲ *An adult pygmy marmoset weighs only about 100 grams*

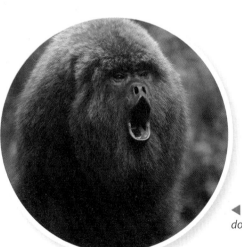

World's Loudest Monkey

How loud can the howler monkeys be? When they shout, you can hear them even from 5 kilometres away! Howler monkeys shout to let others know where their territory is. One group shouts as a call, and in return, the second group answers.

Howler monkeys shout early in the morning and in the evening. They live on treetops and have tails that can grip branches of trees.

◀ *Howler monkeys live in groups where the dominant male has the loudest shout*

▶ *Tarsier babies are the largest as compared to their mothers*

Shy Primates

Tarsiers, with their spooky eyes, are said to bring bad luck by villagers in Borneo. They frighten many with their appearance. These small monkeys are residents of Southeast Asia. Their striking feature is their remarkably huge eyes that they use to see better at night, as they are nocturnal animals. This might be because they lack the tapetum, a reflective layer present in most nocturnal animals, which helps them see in low light. They can rotate their heads 180 degrees and have long ankle bones. They are the only entirely carnivorous primates and they feed on insects, lizards, and snakes.

Sun Soakers

Found in Madagascar and a few neighbouring islands, the ring-tailed lemurs are great sunbathers. Every morning, they sit on the ground with their arms open wide, facing the Sun. These animals live in groups of 15–20.

A ring-tailed lemur has a long, striped, black and white tail. The animals mainly eat fruits. They have powerful scent glands, which they use to mark their territory, communicate, and attack predators.

◀ Ring-tailed lemurs look for food together. After eating, they like to relax in spots that receive sunlight

Close Cousins

Chimpanzees are probably the closest relatives of human beings in the primate family, apart from bonobos. These primate species reside in the tropical forests of Africa and are omnivores. They are extremely intelligent, with logical thinking and problem-solving capabilities. Chimpanzees live in groups called communities and are extroverted by nature. They are known to display love and affection towards others. The mother and child, and siblings share strong bonds and, just like human beings, even they can display a bad temper.

Orangutans

'Orangutan' in Malay means 'person of the forest'. This primate is long-haired, orangish in colour, and has an enormous arm span (almost 7 feet in males) when stretched. Orangutans are found in Sumatra and Borneo.

An average orangutan spends most of its life in trees. It makes itself a bed in the tree by breaking apart branches, twigs, and leaves. It makes a new bed every night, and uses large leaves as an umbrella to keep itself dry from the constant tropical rains.

▼ Orangutans are semi-solitary creatures, which means they like to live around two or three others at a time

⊚ Incredible Individuals

Jane Goodall is a famous British **ethologist**, who has lived among and studied chimpanzees in Gombe on the shores of Lake Tanganyika. She gave us a lot of insights about chimpanzees, such as that they can make tools and perform many social interactions. She has written a number of books and articles on the subject.

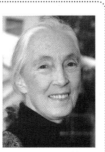

▲ Jane Goodall started her research without a degree

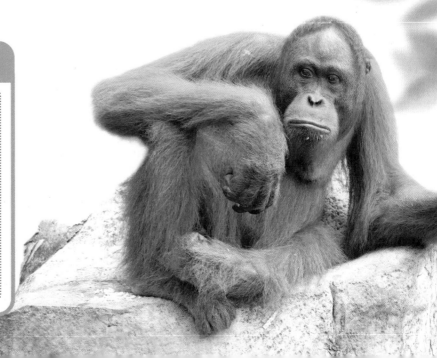

Our Evolution

Do you ever wonder how human beings evolved from apes? Going by the knowledge gained so far, we have discovered that human beings are the most skilled and developed mammals in the history of the evolution of Earth. The story of humans started around six million years ago in Africa. Our primate ancestors spent most of their time on trees, just like modern primates. So, what changed?

🐾 The Rough Details

It is said that an ancient ancestor of human beings came down from the safety of the trees and began to roam the lands—it is not yet certain if they roamed grasslands or forests. It was probably at this point that humans became different from our closest living relatives, the chimpanzees and other such apes.

Scientists have put the human tribe into a group called 'Hominin'. The modern human beings (called *homo sapiens*) are the only living members of this tribe, but fossil evidence shows that many hominins preceded us. The history spans more than a million years:

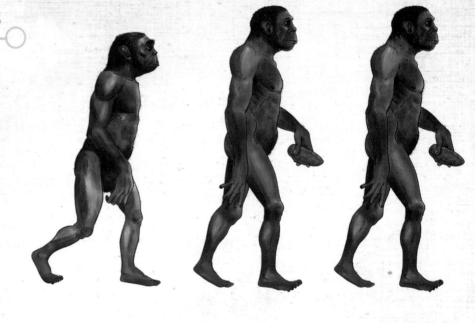

4.4 Million Years Ago

Ardipithecus, so far, is considered the first hominin. While there are ape fossils older than *Ardipithecus,* there is no evidence of them being human ancestors. *Ardipithecus* appeared in forests of present-day Ethiopia. It was probably not a good walker or runner, but its fossils indicate the presence of the same anchors for muscles we have on our pelvis, which chimpanzees and other apes lack.

3 Million Years Ago

Our first true human ancestor, *Australopithecus* appeared in Africa. A female *Australopithecus* was discovered in 1974 in Hadar, Ethiopia. She was named 'Lucy' after a song by the Beatles. The fossil evidence shows that Lucy was a bipedal, which means she walked on two legs. She was seen to have wisdom teeth. *Australopithecus* had a larger and a more complex brain structure.

2 Million Years Ago

Almost 2-million-year-old fossils of *Homo habilis* were discovered in Koobi Fora in Kenya and Olduvai Gorge in Tanzania. The word means 'handy man' or 'hand-using man'. The fossils show that the brain had increased in size and complexity yet again. Scientists feel that *Homo habilis* could use stones as tools. It was the development of such skills that set humans apart in the animal kingdom.

1.7 Million Years Ago

Homo erectus, which refers to the species' relatively erect posture, was the first ancestor to have human-like body proportions. This species first appeared in East Africa and spread to various parts of Africa, Asia, and Europe. Along with the use of stone tools, these early humans discovered fire.

Isn't It Amazing!

Did you know humans are mammals with the longest hair? If you did not cut it, your hair would reach the floor and beyond. Beards and moustaches can also grow very long. A close second is the musk oxen, an animal which lives in the Arctic. It has a long, brown coat which reaches almost down to its feet. The Arctic fox has a thick coat of fur which can survive temperatures that drop below -50° C. Its coat turns from white to brown during the cold harsh winter and even grows longer for more protection.

◀ *History of humankind (L–R: Ardipithecus, Australopithecus, Homo habilis, Home erectus, Homo neanderthalensis, Homo sapiens)*

400,000 Years Ago

Around the time *Homo erectus* was roaming the various continents, a new type of hominin appeared in Europe. They were called *Homo neanderthalensis* or simply Neanderthals, named after the Neander Valley in Germany, where the first fossil was discovered. These are the closest relatives of mankind on the evolutionary map. Their bodies were shorter, and they had larger brains. They also had angular cheek bones and large noses.

Community Living

Neanderthals were the first to exhibit the traits of civilisation. They controlled fire, built shelters, and used stone tools for hunting. They practiced burial rituals for the dead. They were the first to develop art in the form of cave paintings which show their culture, society, and the world they lived in. They disappeared nearly 40,000 years ago. They either assimilated with modern *Homo sapiens* or became extinct.

200,000–100,000 Years Ago

Homo sapiens are thought to have evolved in Africa. The oldest remains unearthed so far are from Morocco. All of us living on planet Earth today belong to this species. *Homo sapiens* have the most complex and largest brain capacities amongst any hominin species. They have an erect posture, light jaws, and small teeth.

Development of Society

Human beings, as they are called, colonised and spread across the different continents on Earth. Our ancestors began the use of complex tools, not just for hunting, but farming as well. They built villages, which created societies. They created art, music, foods, ornaments, clothes, and rituals, which form the basis of human civilisation as we know today.

How Babies Are Born

All living species need to reproduce to survive and exist. Depending upon how the reproduction process takes place, mammals are classified into three main groups—placental, monotremes, and marsupials. The mammals belonging to these three groups also have different ways of nursing their babies.

Placental Mammals

They are the most common mammals in the world as all mammals except monotremes and marsupials are placental. They nourish their unborn babies in the womb through a membrane called **placenta**. The placenta absorbs nutrients and oxygen from the mother's blood. It then passes them onto the foetus through a long cord called the **umbilical cord**. This is the case in most mammals such as tigers, monkeys, elephants, and human beings.

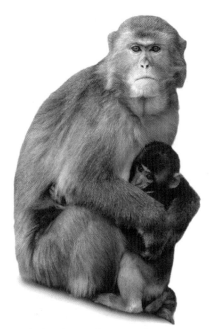

▲ *Monkeys only give birth every couple of years*

Monotremes

Monotremes are the most ancient living order of mammals. The name means 'single hole'. As the name suggests, monotremes have a single opening for excretion and reproduction. They are egg-laying mammals. They have managed to retain certain physical characteristics that were lost in other mammals.

Another interesting feature of monotremes is that they have low body temperatures like reptiles, unlike the other warm-blooded mammals. The platypus and echidnas (spiny anteaters) are monotremes.

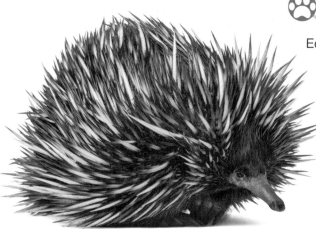

▲ *Echidnas are also known as spiny anteaters*

Echidna

Echidnas can be long-beaked or short-beaked. They are covered in spines and have a tubular beak through which they eat and breathe. They are found in New Guinea and Tasmania, Australia.

The female echidna is followed by many male echidnas during the breeding season. At the end of the gestation period, which is 23 days, the female echidna lays an egg in a skin pouch on her belly. She **incubates** the egg for 10 days until it finally hatches. The baby echidna rests in a burrow and drinks milk from the mother's mammary hairs. Once it develops its fur and spines fully, it can leave the burrow and feed itself.

In Real Life

Research has found that emperor penguins breed on iceshelves. While some breeds live on sea ice, some are found to also live on the iceshelves. As they rely on the ice, the population of emperor penguins could rapidly decline due to global warming. In these harsh and cold conditions, the female emperor penguin produces a single egg. She doesn't build a nest, rather she has the male keep the egg warm.

▶ *An emperor penguin egg weighs around 460 g*

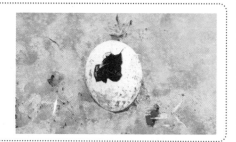

Duck-billed Platypus

Interestingly, the opposite sexes of the duck-billed platypus only interact with each other to mate when they reach the age of four. The mating process takes place in water. The female platypus usually lays two small eggs after a gestation period of two weeks to one month. She incubates the egg for 6–10 days by curling her body around the eggs until her tail touches her bill.

When the eggs hatch, the young platypuses stay in burrows and suckle milk from the mother's mammary hair. People who first began to take notice and observe this animal thought it had a comical appearance, almost like a duck's beak was sewn onto a random mammal. The duck-billed platypus is certainly one of nature's strangest looking animals.

Marsupials

Like placental mammals, marsupials also have placenta but as it is not properly developed, their gestation period is shorter. The animals in this group have a pouch, but do not lay eggs. The females give birth to very tiny and premature babies. These babies stay in the pouch, feeding on the mother's milk until they grow, develop, and are ready for the world. The Tasmanian devil and opossums are examples of marsupials.

Tasmanian Devil

The Tasmanian devil has a short lifespan of eight years. It matures and is ready to mate by the age of two. At one time, a female Tasmanian devil gives birth to two or four young ones. They stop breeding at the age of five. The young ones are bound to the mother or stay in the pouch for 10 months, after which they become independent. They drink milk from the teats in their mother's pouch.

Isn't It Amazing!

The opossum pretends to be dead when it is confronted by a predator! It flops to the ground and rolls its tongue out to the side. It closes its eyes, or makes them look glassy with a vacant, dead stare. It also emits a rancid odour which drives away its predators. Even if its enemy—like a dog or a coyote—decides to jab the motionless body, the opossum remains still. After the predator leaves, the opossum escapes.

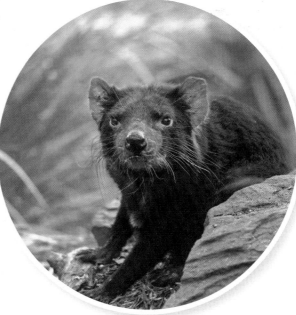

▲ Once the Tasmanian devil was found all over Australia, but now it is only found in Tasmania

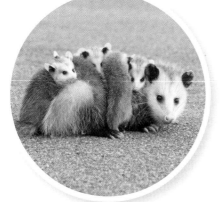

◀ In one week, the birth weight of a baby opossum increases tenfold

Opossum

The male opossum is known to be territorial and violent during the mating season. The gestation period is very short, lasting only 12 days after mating. The opossum gives birth to a litter of 16–20 babies, but less than half of them survive. At birth, they are the size of a mosquito! They are blind for the first two months after birth and stay in the safety of the mother's pouch till 75–85 days. They leave their mother when they are three to four months of age.

◀ Common brushtail possums communicate through sound and scent

From Here to There

Migration is the annual movement of animals from one place to another. Animals migrate for better climatic conditions, food, and for the breeding season. Living in one place could reduce the chances of survival for many animals. It is not just birds and insects that migrate. Quite a few mammals also go through periods of migration.

The Great Migration

Inhabiting the African **savannahs** are the wildebeest. These mammals belong to the antelope family, such as the gazelles. They are known for their annual migration.

Come March, these mammals, with their new calves, leave Serengeti in Tanzania to reach Masai Mara in Kenya. Close to 1.5 million wildebeest travel in an enormous clockwise loop on a year-long trek that spans 1,000 kilometres. They are followed by a few thousand gazelles, impalas and zebras. Scientists are yet to decode the exact reason for this migration; they suspect that a change in the chemical composition of the grass, induced by rains, might be responsible.

In November, they start their trek back to Serengeti. However, the migration is not without its dangers. They not only have to cross rivers filled with crocodiles, but also brave land predators like cheetahs, African dogs, and hyenas. Along the way, they lose approximately 250,000 members.

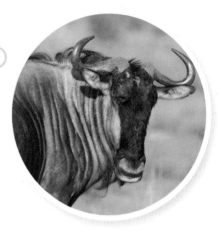

▲ Wildebeest are responsible for the largest terrestrial migration in the world

Oceanic Journey

Humpback whales are mammals living in the oceans. They weigh around 30,000 kilograms. These mammals follow a long-distance migration pattern, travelling close to 10,000 km every year.

In the polar areas where the humpback whales reside, they eat krill in the summer months. However, in winters, when they migrate, breed, and calve, the animals eat nothing. Instead they survive on blubber or fat stored in their bodies. The humpback whales reside in the Northern hemisphere and migrate to Hawaii, while those in the Southern hemisphere migrate to Eastern Australia.

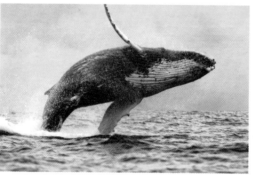

▲ Humpback whales have moved from 'vulnerable' to the 'least concerned' category on IUCN's Red List

▼ Wildebeest seen on the banks of the Mara river, after which the game reserve Masai Mara is named

Isn't It Amazing!

Male humpback whales are great singers. They create songs in the form of high-pitched squeals and whistles or low gurgles. Their songs can last for 30 minutes. It is said that male humpbacks sing to attract mates in the breeding season. They create a new song for each new breeding season, which is picked by many others in the area, making it the 'song of the season'.

Conservation of Endangered Mammals

We share our planet with a variety of flora and fauna, and all species have an equal right to call it home. Apart from that, they make the world we live in beautiful and interesting. They provide for many of our needs; for example we get wool from sheep and milk from cows. Upon visiting a nature park, one thing we all look for are animals. So, is it not our duty to contribute toward saving the animals?

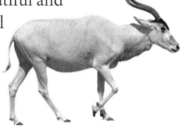

▲ *Many animals form large herds for migration*

🐾 Ways to Help

- Educate people about the importance of animals.

- Make the world in which animals live a better place for them to inhabit. It could be done by cleaning up human waste from their surroundings—removing plastic and other harmful waste thrown around in parks and beaches.

- Volunteer at a zoo, aquarium, or natural reserve in your area.

Let us look at a few animals from around the world which need our help. We may not have seen them if they live in faraway lands. But every animal in this world counts and if they are not conserved, the vast diversity of animals we see might be lost forever.

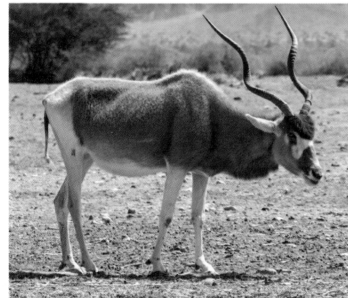

▲ *The Sahara Conservation Fund is active in protecting the addax*

🐾 Lost in the Desert

Addax is a desert antelope known to live in harsh environments. These antelopes are active during nights, since in the daytime they dig into the sand and stay under cover to keep away from the hot desert sun. Once found in abundance around Sahara in Africa, they now live in a confined area between Niger and Chad.

Sadly, this animal is in the Critically Endangered Red List of IUCN. A protected population exists in the Yotvata Hai-Bar Nature Reserve in Israel. Soon, Niger will have a vast area reserved to protect the remaining animals that move in the wild.

The dwindling number of the addax is mainly due to hunting. This mammal's meat and leather are useful commodities purchased by the local people. Droughts and a shrinking habitat also contribute to their endangerment.

🐾 The Spotted Predator

The Asiatic cheetah has long legs, a spotted coat, and a slender frame. It is one of the fastest runners on land. Once upon a time, these animals abounded the Indian sub-continent, Afghanistan, and Central Asia. However, now they fall under the Critically Endangered list of the IUCN. The animals prefer to live in plains and desert-like areas.

Today, their population is concentrated in a remote region of Iran. This reduced population was caused by the loss of prey and hunting activity. The government of Iran is working with various wildlife agencies to create a programme which might save this animal in one of its last reserves.

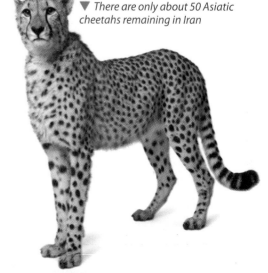

▼ *There are only about 50 Asiatic cheetahs remaining in Iran*

MARINE ANIMALS

HOW IT ALL **BEGAN**

The first fish evolved about 510 million years ago. The evolution of these organisms marks the beginning of complex life which would ultimately result in the evolution of human beings. Fish and marine animals evolved along the same time, dominating the waters of Earth.

The first fish took birth in the oceans and belonged to a class of animals called vertebrates (animals that have backbones). Besides fish, the waters are home to marine animals such as octopuses and sponges. It is important to remember that many marine animals are invertebrates, which means they do not have backbones. Read on to find out some incredible facts about these beings that live under water.

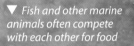
▼ *Fish and other marine animals often compete with each other for food*

The Evolution of Fish

Rewind to 540 million years ago, to a time called the Cambrian Period. Unlike today, the vegetation then was not so evolved or diverse. In fact, the land was inhospitable for life. However, the oceans were bursting with life and this period was called the 'Cambrian Explosion'. The fossil for the first known vertebrate evolved during this period and was called *Haikouichthys ercaicunensis*. The fossil for the earliest primitive **chordate**, called *Pikaia gracilens*, also dates to this period.

Like an Eel

Pikaia gracilens resembled the modern eels. The animal was small, with a tapered, streamlined body. It had eyes, a brain, and a **notochord**. This refers to a flexible, rod-like structure found in the embryos of all vertebrates. It goes on to become a part of the backbone.

▲ *The Pikaia was the first true chordate*

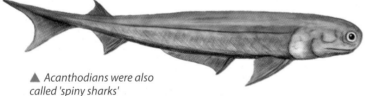

▲ *The extinct lampreys were jawless fish*

Jawless Wonder

You might not recognise the first fish to swim on Earth as they had no jaws or teeth. They began to appear in the Ordovician Period, about 488 million years ago. During this period, Earth looked very different from how it looks today. The ocean covered the area to the north of the tropics and land was limited to a supercontinent called **Gondwana**.

The (now extinct) jawless fish of this period were called ostracoderms. Not more than 30 cm in length, they lived in freshwater and had bony scales which protected the brain. They were bottom feeders, which means they found food on the ocean floor.

The Jaws Emerged

The *Acanthodians* (or spiny shark) were among the first fish with jaws. They emerged in the Silurian Period, about 440 million years ago. During this period, there were large-scale geographical changes due to the melting of giant glaciers. This resulted in a rise in sea levels.

▲ *Acanthodians were also called 'spiny sharks'*

The fish that existed during the Silurian Period survived for about 150–180 million years before they went extinct. Nothing is known about their ancestors, but it is assumed that they originated from the jawless invertebrates.

The *Acanthodians* were small fish with huge eyes and short snouts, indicating that they relied more upon their vision rather than smell. They had bony spines in front of the fins and small, diamond-shaped scales. They had about four fins that they used for manoeuvring rather than locomotion. The latter was managed with the tail.

In Real Life

Sharks are not bony, but **cartilaginous**. Hence, unlike reptiles, mammals, and birds, the skeletons of sharks are made of cartilage and tissue. Human beings also have cartilage in their ears and nose. You might be able to feel it by placing a finger on the tip of your nose. Cartilage has lesser density than bone, and it is more flexible.

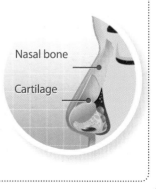

Nasal bone

Cartilage

The Age of the Fish

The period from 420–358 million years ago is called the Devonian Period. It came to be called the 'Age of Fish' because of the variety and wealth of fish that swam in the waters of this period. Among the many species of fish, the placoderms dominated the waters for almost 70 million years, disappearing at the end of the Devonian Period.

The word 'placoderm' means 'plate skin' and as the name suggests, the fish were covered with bony armour, especially around the head and the trunk. The tail was well-developed. The other important features of this fish type were the presence of jaws, with attached tooth-like structures; and the development of well-formed fins at the pectoral and maybe even the pelvic region.

▶ Placoderm were generally small fish, but some could be about 13 feet in length. The Dinichthys is an example of a large placoderm species with a size of about 30 feet

Ancestors of Modern Fish

The earliest shark-like fish appeared in the Devonian Period. They were the first cartilaginous fish to appear, belonging to the group called *Chondrichthyes*. While most of these primitive fish disappeared, few still survived and evolved.

The modern sharks, skates, and ray-fish are cartilaginous fish that originated in the Jurassic Period, about 200 million years ago. During this period, the dry, hot climate changed to subtropical and humid.

The cartilaginous fish had flexible jaws. They could battle with fish that were bigger than themselves. A tail fin helped them swim faster and longer so they could easily pursue their prey.

▶ Helicoprion was another ancient shark. It had a spiral-shaped tooth structure called the tooth-whorl

Whorls

Isn't It Amazing!

Megalodon, meaning 'big tooth', was a huge 25,000 kilogram shark that grew almost 55 feet in length. It had a gaping mouth of 6 feet. Megalodon had sharp teeth which could eat anything, big or small, in the ocean. Each tooth was about 17.7 centimetres in length.
This shark appeared 16 million years ago. It ruled the ocean until two million years ago, when it disappeared. It is now extinct because of extensive changes in the ocean temperatures and lack of prey. But folklore says it still lurks deep in the oceans!

▼ The megalodon is said to be the largest fish that ever swam the waters of our planet

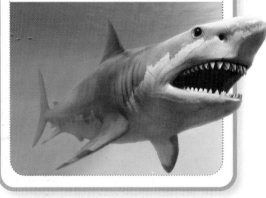

▼ The prehistoric Stethacanthus shark had a strange anvil-shaped dorsal fin on its back. No one knows what it was used for

Anatomy of a Fish

With over 35,000 fish species in the world, scientists have identified important body parts of the animal. These can help distinguish between the various species that swim in the waters of our planet.

Body

Fish have streamlined bodies which help them move smoothly in water. The shape of the body and the tail have evolved in accordance with their habitat. The shape of the body decides a fish's ability to swim. For example, tuna fish are excellent swimmers and have sharp, forked tails that make them agile.

▲ *Most fish have taste buds all over their body*

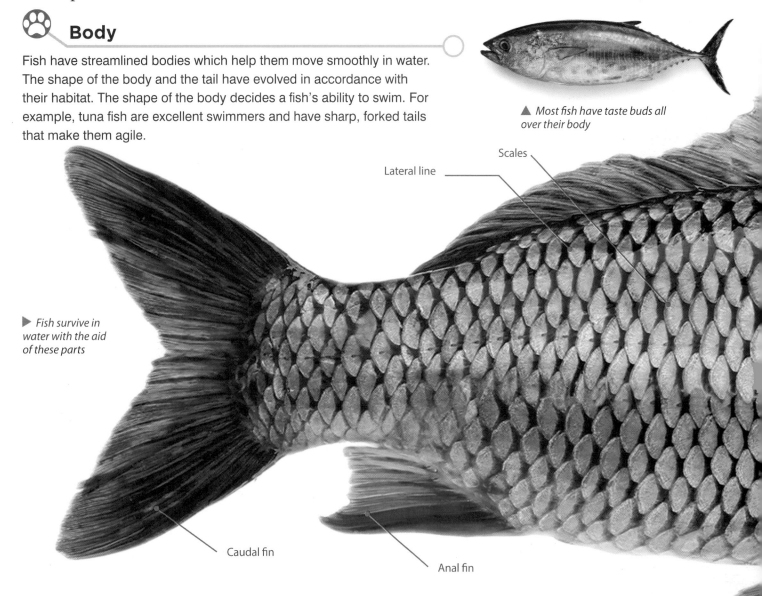

Scales

Lateral line

▶ *Fish survive in water with the aid of these parts*

Caudal fin

Anal fin

Fins

Fish use their fins to swim. The position of the fins on the body determines their functionality. Fish move forward with their tail fins, whereas they use the pectoral fins to swim and balance better. The dorsal fins are used for protection and balance. The ventral and anal fins located on the belly are needed for balance and steering.

Mouth

If a fish has a superior (upward pointing) mouth, it will eat food above it. If a fish has an inferior (downward pointing) mouth, it will eat food from the bottom of the seabed.

Gills

Instead of lungs, fish take in oxygen molecules dissolved in the water through their gills. These are located on both sides of their mouths. They are covered by a series of bones called the operculum. Some fish species have spikes on their gills to protect themselves against predators. Water passes over the tiny network of blood vessels in the gills. The fish force the water to move over the gills using their mouth and throat.

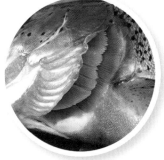

▲ *A close-up of the gills of a fish*

Scales

Most fish have an external covering of scales which act like a protective device. They are unique to fish. Scales come in different sizes and colours; they vary among species and at times even sexes. Like human skin, they protect the fish. The scales are covered by a slimy, mucous layer that protects the fish from bacteria in the water.

Dorsal fins

Lateral Line

Lateral lines are located under the scales of a fish and consist of many tiny openings or holes. These lines run parallel to the fish's body and allow it to feel low vibrations in the water.

Nares

Nares are located on the snouts. They are the two holes that help a fish smell under water. Some fish have a heightened sense of smell because of the nares.

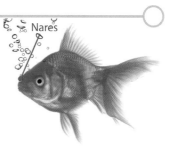

▲ The goldfish have nares which allow them to smell better than human beings

Eye

Nares or nostrils

Mouth

Gill

Gill cover

Pectoral fin

Pelvic fin

Heart

Fish's internal organs such as the stomach, gall bladder, liver, and kidney are similar to mammals. But their hearts are different. While human hearts have four chambers, fish hearts have only two—one chamber receives blood and the other chamber pumps it out.

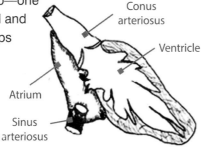

Conus arteriosus

Ventricle

Atrium

Sinus arteriosus

▶ If a fish's blood pressure is too high, it might damage the gills of the fish

Gas Chamber

Most fish do not breathe with their lungs. Instead they have a swim bladder, also called the air bladder. This is a gas-filled sac in their abdominal region. It contains a mixture of oxygen, carbon dioxide, and nitrogen absorbed from the blood. It functions as a **ballast** organ, which means it helps the fish maintain depth without sinking or floating upward. The swim bladder amplifies sound in some fish, like the glass fish. This part is missing in cartilaginous fish, deep-sea dwelling fish, and in a few bony fish.

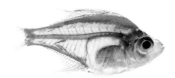

▲ One can clearly see the swim bladder of a glassfish as it is transparent

Fishy Features

The word 'fish' comes from the Old English word 'fisc'. It was used for any animal living in water. To us human beings, from where we stand at the highest position on the evolutionary scale, fish might seem like just another set of animals that cohabit Earth with us. But these forms, which are at the base of the evolutionary scale, have many interesting tales to tell.

Cold-blooded

Fish are **ectotherms** or cold-blooded animals. No, their blood is not cold, as the name suggests. It just means that they cannot regulate their body temperatures internally and rely on external sources such as sunlight or shade to maintain it. Most often, their temperatures tend to be slightly lower than that of the environment to prevent loss of moisture.

Cold-blooded animals use interesting adaptations to overcome the inability to regulate their body temperature. Some species of frogs become **dormant** in the warm weather to prevent moisture loss. Ocean fish stay hydrated by drinking lots of water.

▼ *Goldfish swim in a group called 'school'*

Vertebrates

It is with the fish that the world got its first vertebrates. A vertebrae or backbone supports the body and protects the spinal cord. So, vertebrates need their backbones and brains to survive.

Laying Eggs

Fish lay their eggs in water. However, unlike mammals, birds, and reptiles, they do not lay amniotic eggs, that is, eggs containing **amnion**. Amnion is a fluid-filled sac that keeps the embryos moist.

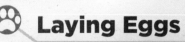

◀ *A siamese female fighting fish guarding her newly laid eggs amongst the bubble nest*

Population of Eggs

Fish lay several eggs at one time. This ensures that the reproduction process is successful. In fish, fertilisation takes place outside the body. In most cases, the fertilised eggs are not looked after by the adults. This exposes the eggs to predators and other dangers that could reduce the number of eggs drastically. So, not all eggs lead to successful reproduction. Those that fail to hatch are recycled into the ecosystem.

💡 Isn't It Amazing!

A unique feature of the clownfish is that they are all born male during birth. If their group is missing a dominant female, one clownfish will change its sex. They cannot change back to male. This is because a school of clownfish follows a hierarchy. The most dominant female rules the school. So, if there is no dominant female, the dominant male changes sex. Similarly, moray eels and gobies also change sex.

A History of Jawless Fish

There are so many fish on this planet. Even within the same species, there is a great diversity. For example, though the hammerhead shark and tiger shark belong to the same species, they look quite different. So, in order to study fish, scientists have classified them into three broad groups according to their features. These groups are the jawless fish, cartilaginous fish, and bony fish.

Primitive Jawless Fish

Agnathans comprise the early species of jawless fish. This includes lampreys, hagfish and other extinct groups of fish. The core identifiers of these fish are the absence of jaws, paired fins, pelvic fins, and vertebral columns. They have slimy skin and a cartilaginous skeleton, instead of a bony skeleton. They also have a light-sensitive pineal gland. For the agnathans, reproduction and development are external. There is no known form of post-natal care. Some fish show the first vertebral column in their bodies, known as the notochord. They retain the notochord for the rest of their lives.

Jawless Fish

The two main types of jawless fish were the lampreys and the hagfish. They had unpaired fins and circular mouths. Their heart had two chambers and they were ectothermic in nature. It is uncertain if jawless fish lived in shallow, marine waters, or if the force of the freshwater streams washed their fossils towards shallow water streams.

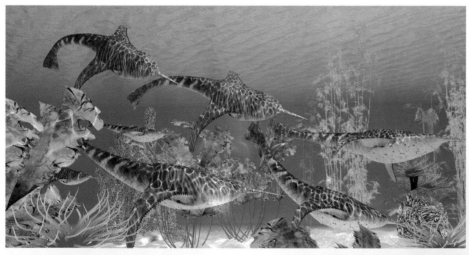

▲ *Devonian Doryaspis fish; Doryaspis is an extinct genus of primitive jawless fish that lived in the ocean during the Devonian Period*

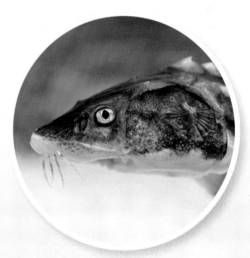

▲ *Biologists say that sturgeon fish are the most primitive of the bony fish alive today*

Feeding Habits of Agnathans

Since they are ectothermic, or cold-blooded, they eat little food and do not rely on a speedy metabolism to stay warm. The early jawless fish were soft-bodied. They fed on tiny organisms by the process of filter-feeding. Fish would prey on microorganisms at the bottom of the sea by sucking or nibbling from their mouths. The food would then be passed onto their large gill cavities, which also processed water and helped the fish breathe.

The gill cavities had very large surface areas to suit this purpose, and the gill apparatus would redirect the food to the canal. The gill, therefore, evolved to be multipurpose and took care of the eating and breathing needs of the fish. The head and gills were protected by a dermal armour, whereas their tails had unrestricted freedom of movement.

▲ *Sharks are cartilaginous fish*

Lampreys and Hagfish

These fish have interested evolutionary scientists because modern agnathans continue to possess primitive characteristics. This order also includes the oldest known craniate fossils. Lampreys and hagfish are modern agnathans.

🐾 Lampreys

Lampreys and hagfish have the notochord. It is a circular, jawless mouth. Lampreys also have unpaired fins and eel-like scaleless skin. They have one or two dorsal fins, well-developed eyes, and teeth on their tongue, as well as an oral disc. Adult lampreys are sized between 35–60 centimetres. They also have an elongated larval stage. They breed in freshwater rivers, lakes, and ponds. This makes them **anadromous**, which means they migrate up from rivers to spawn in the sea.

▶ *A lamprey has 7 gill pores on each side of the head*

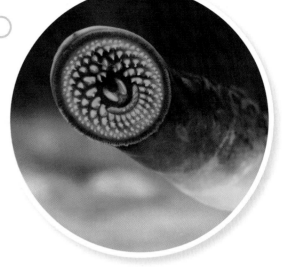

▲ *Some species of lampreys can be parasitic as they feed on the blood of other fish*

🐾 Reproduction in Lampreys

When lampreys reproduce, they build a nest in the water, lay their eggs, and die after fertilisation. Their breeding period can last for 18 months. The larvae grow to a maximum size of 10 centimetres. There are 41 extant species of lampreys, out of which 18 are parasitic and 23 remain confined to freshwater habitats. They also exist in the ocean but prefer coastal regions. They are found in most temperate regions, with the exception of Africa. They are not tolerant of high water temperatures, and thus do not thrive in tropical environments. The landlocked lampreys are limited in size.

🐾 Reproduction in Hagfish

Hagfish usually inhabit high-saline waters and do not like direct exposure to light. Thus, they are found at the mouths of rivers or more than 1,000 metres below the ocean's surface. They are the only vertebrate whose body fluids are isosmotic with seawater and they are found only in marine waters. Their diets consist of dead fish and invertebrates. Like scavengers, they eat the insides of dying fish. They cannot directly penetrate the skin of their prey, so they enter natural openings such as the prey's mouth, gills, or anus. They do not have jaws, but instead have a pair of tooth-like projections that help pull up food. They do not primarily prey on fish and are themselves often consumed by seabirds and crustaceans. They have a very slow metabolism and only need to feed a few times in one month.

◀ *As opposed to lampreys, hagfish do not have a larval stage*

🐾 Hagfish

Hagfish belong to the order Myxiniformes. They are known for their eel-like bodies. A fossil study of hagfish shows that their anatomies have remained unchanged for the past 300 million years! Their bodies are scaleless and they have unpaired fins, a single nostril, and paddle-like tails. They can be found in a range of colours from pink to blue-grey. Their teeth are located on their tongues, and they have degenerate eyes. On an average, they measure about 50 centimetres. Each hagfish has both the ovaries and the testes, but only one functional gonad.

👆 In Real Life

An adult hagfish can secrete so much slime that it can turn a big bucket of water into thick gel within minutes. When held by the tail, the hagfish escapes by secreting a slime that becomes a thick gel when in contact with water. They clean themselves of this slime by tying themselves into an overhand knot and using it to scrape themselves from head to tail.

Bony v/s Cartilaginous Fish

A distinct feature of the fish evolution cycle was the early development of bone, cartilage, and enamel-like substance. This helped the fish adapt to diverse aquatic environments in the water and even on land.

🐾 Differences

There are many differences between the bony fish and the cartilaginous fish. The most important difference is that the skeleton of the bony fish is made of bones, whereas the skeleton of cartilaginous fish is made of cartilage.

Features	Bony Fish	Cartilaginous Fish
Skeleton	The **endoskeleton** is made of bones. Their **exoskeleton** or external covering is made of cycloids (thin, bony plates).	The endoskeleton is made of cartilage. Their exoskeleton is made of placoid, that are small denticles with a sharp, enamel coating.
Mouth	They have an anterior tip mouth opening.	They have a ventral mouth.
Operculum	They have opercula on either side of the gills.	They do not have an operculum.
Tail	They have a homocercal tail fin.	They have a heterocercal tail fin.
Swim bladder	Also called an air bladder or buoyancy organ, it is present in most bony fish. It contains oxygen and allows the fish to maintain their depth without floating upwards or sinking.	It is absent in all cartilaginous fish and bottom-dwelling fish.
Habitat	They are found in both freshwater and marine water.	They are predominantly present in marine waters.
Reproduction	They externally fertilise their eggs.	The fertilisation is internal.
Excretion	They excrete ammonia.	They excrete urea.

🐾 Flying Fish

The flying fish is a bony fish commonly found in warm seas. They consume a variety of small creatures, but mainly plankton and measure 17–30 centimetres in length. These fish have pectoral fins that are like a bird's wings. They use these fins to easily glide over water. They usually swim in schools and consist of over 40 different types of oceanic fish. Some species such as the blue flying fish have two wings, whereas some are four-winged, like the California flying fish. They are preyed on by dolphins, tuna, and mackerel. They avoid these predators with their aerial skills.

▲ *Illustration of the flying fish*

Flying fish do not generally fly, but rather glide on their fins at the speed of about 59 kmph. They can easily cover a distance of 200 metres. The flying fish build up speed under water, then become airborne, making many consecutive glides with their tails propelling their movement above water. The strong fliers can even go as fast as around 400 metres in one single glide!

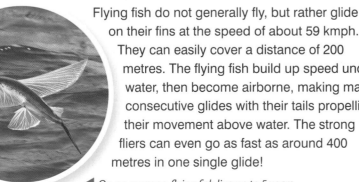

◀ *On an average, flying fish live up to 5 years*

🐾 Dogfish

Dogfish is an example of a cartilaginous fish. It travels in a dense school of fish and preys on other fish and invertebrates. The spiny shark has a sharp spine in front of each of its two dorsal fins. The dorsal fins have venom glands that can cause painful injuries. It is between 60–140 centimetres long. People kill dogfish for food or to produce shark liver oil. They have also been used to make fertilisers.

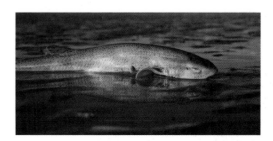

▲ *Dogfish have been considered a nuisance because they end up ripping fishnets after taking bait*

Predatory Sharks

Sharks—for some, hearing the word itself sends chills down the spine. In reality, most sharks do not attack humans unless they feel threatened. However, human beings hunt sharks for their fins, teeth, meat, and skin. So human beings do pose a threat to their survival. There are over 500 species of sharks in the world today.

 ## Behaviour and Intelligence

Although considered to be instinct-driven hunters, many species of sharks have exhibited complex problem-solving skills and high curiosity. They have also shown signs of playful behaviour by repeatedly rolling around in kelp and chasing a trail in the ocean for fun. If a shark feels threatened, it exhibits exaggerated swimming movements to ward off predators. The intensity of the movements is directly dependent on how threatened the shark feels.

Sleep Patterns

Some sharks sleep like dolphins, with one part of their brain active and awake, while the rest of the brain rests. Some sharks use their spiracles to continue swimming while they sleep. Their spinal cord coordinates the activity of swimming so that the brain can rest. Some sink to the bottom of the ocean and lie still with their eyes open and actively pump water over their gills.

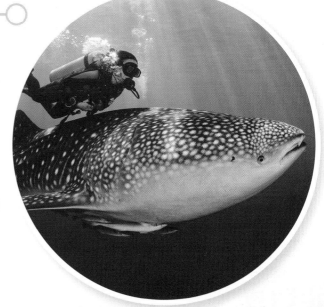

▲ A scuba diver is seen swimming with the whale shark. These sharks are harmless, but they can be spooked by too much movement or artificial light

▶ There are 10 different species of hammerhead sharks. They vary in size but have the same basic features

Hammerhead Sharks

Hammerhead sharks are cartilaginous animals. Each hammerhead shark is 13–20 feet in length and weighs anywhere between 230 and 450 kilograms. What makes this shark unique is the shape of its head, which looks like a flattened hammer. With this peculiar shape, the hammerhead shark can lift and turn its head quickly.

Their wide-set eyes give them a wider view of the surroundings. The hammerhead sharks have expanded nostrils, thereby giving them a better sense of smell and better ability to locate the prey than other fish. Moreover, the underside of the wide head has **electroreceptive organs**, which help these sharks detect the electrical impulses given off by their prey. Great hammerhead sharks are greyish brown or olive green on top, with a white underside.

▲ *The scalloped hammerhead shark has been listed as Critically Endangered due to overfishing for its fins*

Hunting

The great hammerhead is the largest of the 10 identified species of this shark. It has sharp, blade-like teeth. It preys on larger fish, squids, crabs, smaller sharks, and its favourite, the stingrays. As a matter of fact, the shark uses its electroreceptive organs to hunt for stingrays, which usually bury themselves under sand. They use their enormous heads to hold the stingrays down during a fight.

Habitat

The sharks are present in tropic or temperate marine waters. They feed around shallow coastal areas, estuaries, and salty waters. In winters, huge schools of hammerhead sharks are seen migrating towards the warmth of the equator and in summer they move towards the poles.

Young Ones

All species of hammerhead sharks are viviparous, which means that the females retain fertilised eggs within their bodies to give birth to live young ones. The female great hammerhead shark gives birth to several dozens of young ones at a time. The females give birth in shallow waters in summer and spring. The young ones continue to stay there until they are old enough to venture into the oceans.

▶ *Sharks have been around for more than 400 million years*

The True Eels

Eels belong to the order Anguilliformes and are known as teleost fish. The most famous types of eels are the common freshwater eels and aggressive marine morays.

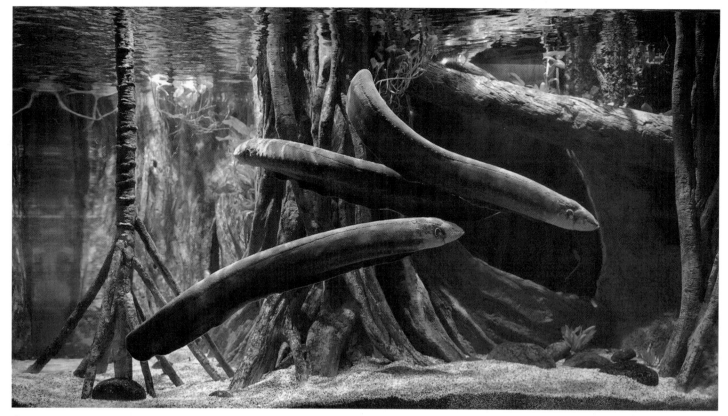

▲ *A group of electric eels swimming together in an aquarium*

🐾 Life as an Eel

Eels are known for their elongated, wormlike bodies and characterised by the absence of pelvic fins (fins on the bottom of the body) and scales that are usually found in other fish families. Almost all eels are found in marine (saltwater) habitats with an interesting exception being the freshwater eel. Even though this eel lives in freshwater rivers and lakes, it travels to a marine environment to spawn, and the young eels then travel back to the freshwater. This phenomenon makes the freshwater eels **catadromous**.

The name 'eel' has been applied to species of different orders as well. Some examples are electric eels, bobtail snipe eels, swamp eels, and spiny eels. However, 'true eels' belong to the order Anguilliformes. These animals have made a significant contribution to the ecosystems. In food chains, they are predators of other fish and invertebrates such as molluscs and crustaceans. Eels have also become a delicacy in many parts of the world.

🐾 Appearance

Eels vary in size according to their species. They range from 10 cm to 3 m in length and can weigh more than 65 kg. The conger eel is the largest in the eel family, reaching 3 m in length. An adult conger eel weighs around 110 kg.

🐾 Social Behaviour

Eels often live in groups in individual holes called eel pits, with only certain species such as the electric eel living in solitary conditions. These pits are found in shallow waters or in the bottom layer of the ocean. Some eels adapt to deeper waters and reach depths of 4,000 metres. Other eels are active swimmers and remain approximately 500 metres below the surface.

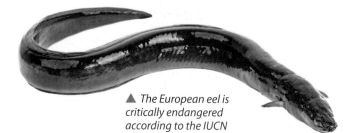

▲ *The European eel is critically endangered according to the IUCN*

Eels and Human Beings

Different species of eels are used as food in different parts of the world. Even though raw eel blood is toxic to human beings, the toxins are neutralised while cooking. The most commonly known culinary use of eel is seen in Japanese food. Freshwater eels are known as unagi and marine eels are known as anago. Jellied eels are a tradition in London and eels from the Comacchio area, in Italy, are a speciality. Eels are also often used for entertainment. In the USA, moray eels are widely used in tropical saltwater aquariums.

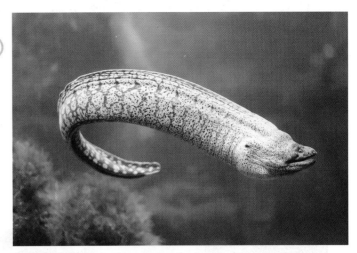

▲ Though there are many species of eels present in water, there is a specific type of eel used in different cuisines

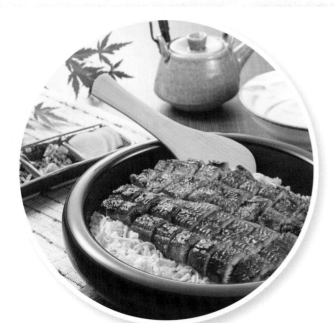

▲ Kabayaki is a dish prepared in Japanese cuisine. It is made with an unagi eel. The dish has different methods of preparation

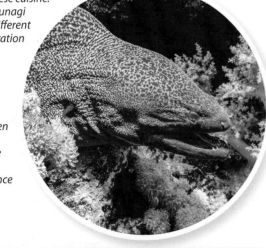

▶ It is easy to distinguish between other eels and the moray eel because of its drastically different appearance

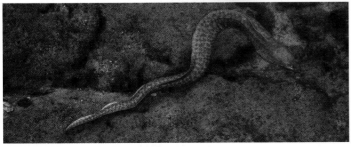

▲ An eel is seen moving on dead patch reefs. These provide shelter to eels

Moray Eels

Moray eels are seen around the world. There are 200 species of these eels found in the oceans and seas. Most of the species are seen in brackish waters; only some prefer freshwater. So, these eels are found in both freshwater and saltwater habitats.

The moray eels living in tropical climates live in coral rubble rocks, dead patch reefs, and coral reefs. They are located near the equator. The reason that these eels have long bodies is that they have more vertebrae. Unlike in other eels, the moray eels have vertebrae between the pre-tail and tail regions of their bodies. They are carnivorous animals who attack and eat cuttlefish, barracudas, groupers, octopuses, and sea snakes.

⊙ Incredible Individuals

Alexander von Humboldt (1769–1859) was a naturalist from Germany. For some reason, he set out in search of some electric eels while he was travelling in South America. He asked some people to help him catch electric eels that were at least 2 metres in length. Surprisingly, they made around 30 horses charge into the water. The surprised eels jumped out of the water and sent shocks through the horses in defence. Once they were tired out, the men collected the eels and provided them to Humboldt. He then wrote about the incident of the 'jumping' electric eels.

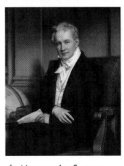

▲ He was the first to connect altitude sickness to a lack of oxygen

Skates and Ratfish

Skates and ratfish are cartilaginous fish. They are related to the shark family, but their appearances vary greatly.

Skates

Skates are very interesting-looking marine animals that belong to the order Rajiformes. They have enlarged pectoral fins that extend from the snout to the base of the tail. Typically, skates have two dorsal fins and their mouth and gills are located in the bottom section of their bodies. They have sharp noses and solid or patterned coats. Skates can vary in size according to their species. The common skate can reach up to 2.8 metres, while the little skate is just 50 centimetres long.

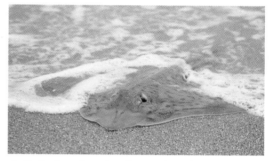

▶ *Skates should not be confused with stingrays*

Features of Skates

Skates inhabit oceans all around the world, from the Arctic to the Antarctic waters. They are benthic, which means that they are found partially buried in the bottom of the ocean. They are very graceful swimmers. They are carnivores and prey aerially on fish, molluscs, and crustaceans. Skates have very low reproductive rates and lay eggs. Their eggs are popularly called 'mermaid's purse' because they are found ashore and are protected by a leathery capsule-like case. In 2006, they were named as a critically endangered species by the IUCN.

▲ *Skates have been in existence since the Jurassic period*

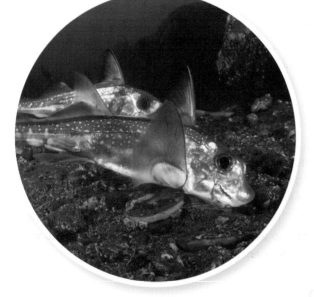

▲ *Ratfish's swim is often termed as aquatic flight due to its resemblance to a bird*

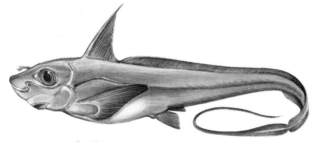

▲ *Chimaera monstrosa are commonly known as rabbit fish or ratfish*

Ratfish

Ratfish, also known as chimaera, belong to the subclass Holocephali, class Chondrichthyes and are related to the well-feared sharks. They are scaleless and are sized between 0.3-1.2 metres in length. They have projecting snouts, ventral mouths, large pectoral and pelvic fins, and very large eyes. They have two dorsal fins that are fronted with poisonous glands. They also have a sharp spine and large, wing-like pectoral fins. Their coats can be of a range of silvery to blackish colours. Like rats, they have slender tails, a prominent feature after which they have been named.

Features of Ratfish

Ratfish are found in temperate or cold waters in diverse marine habitats. They are not agile swimmers, which makes them an easy target for predators. Ratfish feed on small fish, molluscs, and crustaceans. They use their strong teeth to grind their prey. When ratfish reproduce, their females lay eggs that are protected by sharp coverings. These fish are hunted because they are edible and considered to be delicious. They are also killed for the liver oil they produce, which is used as a lubricant for guns and other such instruments.

The Unique Swordfish

Swordfish are large ocean fish. Their distinctive feature is their long flat bill, which bears a close resemblance to a sword, therefore awarding them the nomenclature of swordfish or broadbill.

Appearance

They are elongated, scaleless fish with a tall dorsal fin. They use their long snout to slash at their prey. The 'sword' is flat, rather than rounded as in marlins. Marlins and swordfish belong to the same family along with other spear-nosed fish. The bodies of swordfish are very large, known to grow up to the length of about 4.6 metres. They can weigh about 650 kilograms. They have a distinctive purplish or bluish coat on the top which blends into a silvery and white coat near the underside. So they can blend in well near the surface of the water as well as with what is found living below them. The swordfish is also distinguished by its lack of pelvic fins and teeth.

Swordfish are incapable of maintaining a body temperature higher than the temperature of the surrounding waters. Instead, they have unique muscle and brown tissue that warms blood flowing to the brain and eyes, enabling them to tolerate the extreme cold of the ocean's depths. This is what gives them the sharp eyesight that proves fundamental to their survival at various stages.

▶ The blue marlin swordfish is one of 12 species

Social Behaviour

Swordfish are isolated fish and they do not form schools; but they look for food with the others in a group. They are often sighted near the surface of the water engaging in an activity called 'breaching', where they are seen jumping out of the water. They are one of the fastest animals in the ocean, moving at a speed of 80 kmph. This affords them a significant advantage over their prey. The prey mostly consists of fish such as rockfish, the barracuda, and molluscs such as squids. They possess an enormous appetite owing to their size and are known to hunt actively at night. In the case of swordfish, conception is an external process where the female releases eggs into the open ocean and the male secretes sperm, leading to fertilisation.

◀ From the fertilised eggs, swordfish hatch as larvae. They are 4 millimetres in length

Migration

Though they are found at various depths in the ocean, swordfish are known to migrate through warm and cold waters depending on the season. They tend to stick to warmer waters. The majority of them are found in the Pacific Ocean. They tend to migrate a great deal in order to find food and to be able to stay in the warmer areas of the water. They also go back to cooler waters in the summer to avoid getting too hot. Ideally, they want water that is between 17–21°C.

Current State

Swordfish have few predators. These include human beings, large sharks, and killer whales. Their numbers have always faced the highest threat from human beings. The start of the century had seen a threat to the existence of swordfish because of the popularity and demand for it at restaurants. The IUCN took notice and started working on curbing the rapid decline of the swordfish population.

The Smooth Rays

Rays are the closest relatives of sharks. There are 600 odd species of these fish, the most famous being the stingrays. The eagle ray, the mobula ray, the blue-spotted ray, and the manta ray are some other species.

Body Type

Stingrays have flat bodies that look wide due to the fact that their fins extend to both extremities of their bodies from head to trunk. Their bodies are supported by cartilage instead of bones, just like their shark relatives. They defend themselves with their tails, which have jagged edges and long spines on them. Some stingrays even carry a dangerous venom in their tails.

▶ The stingrays have an average lifespan of 20 years

Habitat

Stingrays inhabit shallow, warm temperate and tropical waters around the world. They prefer staying partially buried in the sand on the ocean floor; it keeps them safe from predators. These patient fish also stay buried waiting for their prey to swim by, so they might catch them. Stingrays eat mussels, oysters, crabs, and shrimps, which they crush with their jaws.

Deadly Stingrays

Most stingrays swim by moving their entire body in a wave, which propels them forward. If one happened to step onto a stingray, it would lash at them with its tail, causing deadly wounds. Some human beings have even died during such accidents. If you want to avoid stepping on a stingray, just move your feet quickly in a shuffling motion. These movements will cause vibrations that can alert the stingrays to back off.

Young Ones

Stingrays are ovoviviparous, which means the young ones are hatched from eggs held within the female's body. Females give birth once a year to 2–6 young ones at a time. The offspring are fully developed within the mother's body, so they look developed when born, ready to lead independent lives.

Senses

The mouth, nostrils, and gills are located on the underside of the stingray, while its eyes are on the top. Scientists believe that the eyes do not help them much in hunting, but they have special sensors which help them detect electric charges emitted by the prey they are hunting.

Freshwater v/s Saltwater

Fish have been in existence for more than 450 million years. They have repeatedly evolved to fit into almost every conceivable type of aquatic habitat. The general idea of a fish can often be misleading as there are over 30,000 species of fish and their shapes and structures vary drastically.

 ## Habitat

Fish inhabit two broad types of habitats. They are the freshwater and saltwater habitats. Marine habitats can be divided into deep ocean floors (benthic), mid-water oceanic (bathypelagic), surface oceanic (pelagic), rocky coast, sandy coast, muddy shores, bays, estuaries, and others. Current human knowledge is limited to their geographical distribution and not the origin of said distribution.

Types of Freshwater Fish

Freshwater fish have been classified as warm-water, cool-water and cold-water. Catfish are warm-water fish who like the water to be around 27° C in temperature.

Perch and walleye prefer cool water, with an average temperature of 16° C to 27° C, while cold-water fish such as trout prefer low temperatures between 10°C to 16°C.

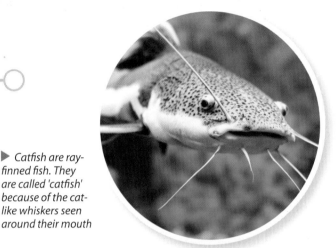

▶ *Catfish are ray-finned fish. They are called 'catfish' because of the cat-like whiskers seen around their mouth*

Types of Saltwater Fish

From the fossils collected over the years, palaeontologists have classified saltwater fish into three categories—Agnatha, Chondrichthyes, and Osteichthyes.

Order Agnatha refers to a type of jawless fish having a circular mouth with rings of teeth. Hagfish and lampreys are the two types of agnathans.

Order Chondrichthyes consists of sharks and stingrays. We can trace their origin to the Jurassic Era, about 200 million years ago.

Order Osteichthyes consists of bony fish. These are the most common type of fish, with over 23,000 species belonging to this order.

▲ *Fish can also drown when there is a lack of oxygen in the water*

How Fish Choose Their Habitats

How is it that some fish prefer freshwater habitats and others prefer saltwater habitats? Fish prefer habitats that provide opportunities for mating, plenty of food, and have few predators. There is another factor that affects their choice of habitats. It is the salinity of the water.

Freshwater fish can survive in salt-deficient waters. In fact, they have developed certain physiological mechanisms that allow them to concentrate salts within their own bodies in the freshwater habitats. Saltwater fish, on the other hand, excrete salts. But the few fish that can live in both habitats have developed various mechanisms to deal with the differences between the two.

The Ferocious Piranhas

Piranhas have a very nasty reputation among human beings. People believe that they can bite or attack people in groups. This is because of incorrect portrayals in movies. Though piranhas can be fierce and fearsome, there are very few reports of them actually biting human beings.

🐾 Species

There are 20 confirmed species of piranhas living in South America. They are freshwater fish found in rivers and lakes. Among them, the black piranha is the largest. It follows a carnivorous diet. Other species, like the red-bellied piranha, follow an omnivorous diet.

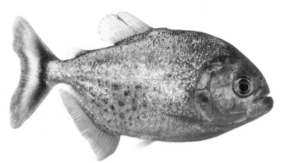

▲ *Red-bellied piranha are sometimes kept as aquarium fish*

🐾 Behaviour

Piranhas are often seen swimming in groups as this is the best way to protect themselves from predators. When they feel threatened, they warn their enemies to leave them alone by 'barking'. They only bite when the attacker continues to annoy them. They feed on small shrimps, worms, and even molluscs. Once it sees a prey, a piranha will swim closer to it and open its mouth wide. Inside its mouth, it has triangle-shaped teeth. They are extremely sharp. A piranha can open up its mouth and gobble up smaller shrimps or molluscs in one quick gulp! Schools of piranhas can contain around 100 individuals. Each piranha can grow to 35 centimetres in size.

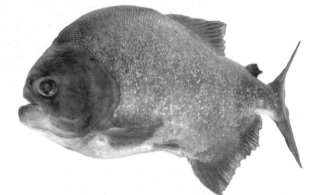

▲ *Black-bellied piranha piranhas can bite with a force three times their own body weight*

▼ *The red-bellied piranhas are typically found in white water rivers such as the Amazon River Basin*

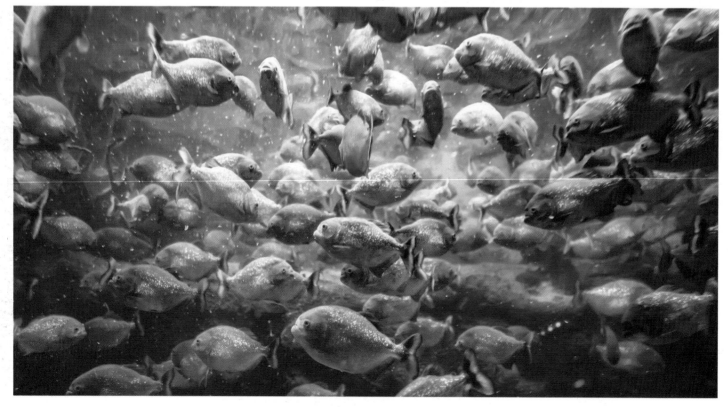

A Poisonous Defence

Whether they live in the ocean or a large aquarium, fish make the world beautiful. They are also great at defending themselves against predators. Quite a few of these creatures have defence mechanisms that could harm not just their predators, but also human beings.

🐾 Sting like a Stonefish

A stonefish is about 30 centimetres in length, with a large head and mouth, and small eyes. These details sound ordinary, but the fish is extraordinary. It carries venom in its skin and in sacs attached to the razor-sharp spines along its back.

When attacked or accidentally stepped onto, the stonefish pushes the spines into the predator and releases the poison. The sting of the spine can lead to paralysis or even death in a few cases. These fish are bottom-dwellers; they live in estuaries, rocks, or in the corals found in the world's oceans.

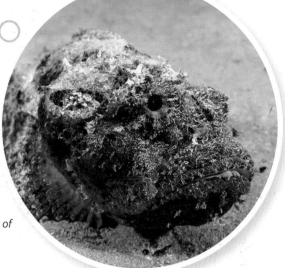

▶ *A stonefish uses the rocks and corals of its surroundings as camouflage*

🐾 All Puffed Up

Pufferfish, also known as blowfish, have the amazing ability to expand. They swim clumsily, making them an easy target for predators. But to escape, the fish fill their elastic stomach with water, and at times air, to become an inedible ball several times larger than their size. Some species of pufferfish have spines on them, making them even less palatable.

The next line of defence the pufferfish uses is tetrodotoxin, a deadly toxin present in almost all 120 species of pufferfish. It is so lethal that the predators, including humans, barely stand a chance for survival. There is enough poison in a single pufferfish to kill almost 30 adult human beings. There is no **antidote** available to fight the toxin.

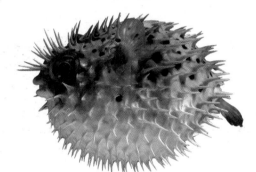

▲ *The only species immune to pufferfish toxin are sharks*

🐾 Fatal Red

The average length of a red lionfish is about one foot. It lives amongst the rocks and crevices of the Indian Ocean and the Pacific Ocean, but it has been introduced to warm waters worldwide. The red lionfish looks striking with brown, red, and white stripes.

It has around 18 venom-filled, needle-shaped dorsal fins. If disturbed, it spreads its fins and if further intimidated, it attacks. If a human being is attacked by the sting of the red lionfish, they might feel nauseous and would not be able to tolerate the pain, but it is rarely fatal.

◀ *The red lionfish is a prized aquarium fish*

The King Salmon

Chinook salmon, or the king salmon, are the largest of the salmon species found in the Pacific. They can grow up to almost 3 feet in length. They live in the cold waters of the upper reaches of the Pacific Ocean in countries such as the United States of America and Canada. Chinook salmon can be found even in Russia and Japan.

A Dual Life

Chinook salmon are **anadromous** fish, which means they can live in freshwater as well as the salty ocean waters. Their life cycle starts and ends in freshwater. They spend their early years in the ocean as they can eat plenty of food and thrive in the open waters.

▲ When Chinook salmon swim upstream for spawning, they often become food for grizzly bears

▶ Chinook salmon are blue-green on the head and back, and silver on the sides. They change colour when moving to freshwater. During the mating season, both male and female Chinook salmon display a slight shade of red on the tail and fins

Eggs

The process of reproduction begins when the Chinook salmon migrate to their breeding grounds. The female digs a small hole in the sandy bottom of a freshwater river or stream. This is like a nest and is called redd. This is where the eggs are laid. A Chinook salmon can lay about 1,000 eggs at one time.

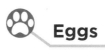

▲ These fish hatch in freshwater but spend their adult lives at sea

The eggs laid by the female are fertilised by the male salmon. Both guard the eggs from predators. The eggs stay put until the embryo develops. These salmon spend so much energy on travelling to the breeding grounds and protecting the eggs that they die even before the eggs can hatch.

Alevins

On complete development, the embryo spins inside the egg until it hatches, after which the babies are released. These baby salmon are called **alevins**. The alevins stay near the nest. They have a yolk sac attached to themselves. They take their nourishment from there and grow. They continue to do so until they learn to find their own food.

Fry

Once the fish finish feeding from the yolk sac and grow, they move from the nest. The baby salmon without the yolk sac are called the fry. The fry leave the nest and move to the surface of the water. They continue to live in the freshwater until they are ready to move to the sea.

The amount of time spent by the fry varies amongst different species of salmon. Chinook fry spend less than five months in freshwater. They keep themselves safe by hiding behind boulders and logs.

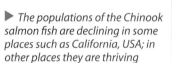
▶ The populations of the Chinook salmon fish are declining in some places such as California, USA; in other places they are thriving

Smolt

At this stage, the fry is big enough to move towards the ocean. The fish continues to grow. The face, jaw and scales are much larger now. Their bodies become long, elongated and silvery in a process called smolting.

The smolts continue to grow as they move towards the estuary. Here they get a mix of fresh and salty water, helping them adjust to the presence of salt. They feed to grow and survive in the ocean.

Open Waters

The Chinook salmon can spend up to eight years in sea water. They are then ready to migrate back to the stream where they were born. This is what makes the life cycle of salmon so interesting. All species of salmon, including Chinooks, swim against the tide and move upstream to complete their goal of laying and fertilising eggs in their original homes. It is said that the chemicals released by their bodies help them adapt to these changing environments of freshwater and salty water.

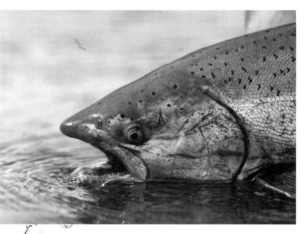

Isn't It Amazing!

Did you know we can trace hiccups back to our 'fishy roots'? A hiccup happens due to a spasm of the diaphragm and is followed by an involuntary gulp. Originally, for fish, breathing was a process involving the brain, throat, and gills. In human beings, the process includes the throat, the chest, and the diaphragm, and sometimes, this complex arrangement can spasm our nerves, resulting in a hiccup! Once we begin to hiccup, it is kept going by a motor reflex seen in ancient tadpoles. It helped them direct water only to their gills, but is not useful for us. However, it does shed some light on our common ancestry.

Full Circle

If not eaten by bears and other predators, the salmon will safely reach home. There, once again, like their parents, they will lay eggs and fertilise them. During the journey, the salmon rely on their surroundings, the sun, and scents to reach their destination.

Hooked noses on the males help them fight others so that they can win over a female and mate with her. The females lay eggs in the redd, which they form by pushing aside small rocks.

Portuguese Man O' War

This interesting-sounding animal gets its name from its uppermost part, which sits above water and resembles a Portuguese sailing warship at full sail. It is also called Floating Terror. Let us take a look at this creature that is often wrongly thought to be a jellyfish.

🐾 Full Blown Sail

The Portuguese man o' war is about three metres long. It has tentacles which can reach a massive length of almost 50 metres. It is found in warm oceanic waters around the world. The Portuguese man o' war is a cousin of the jellyfish. It is an interesting animal. It appears to be a single organism, but in reality, it is a colony of hundreds of hydra-like individuals. These are called polyps and they work in perfect tandem.

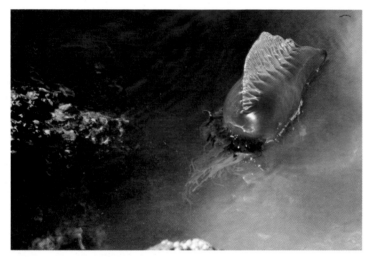

▲ The Portuguese man o' war has a beautiful shape and colour, but you should not approach it as it can sting you

🐾 Polyps

The polyps are divided into four types based on the functions they perform. The uppermost polyp is the float polyp, and gives the organism its unique name. It is a gas-filled chamber and is also known as pneumatophore.

A man o' war simply moves with the oceanic currents. If it feels threatened, the float polyp deflates to submerge for a short while.

The next are the tentacles or the dactylozooids, also known as the stinging polyps. They are covered with poison-filled cells called nematocysts, which paralyse and kill fish and other small marine creatures. Man o' war is not fatal to humans but can cause a sting that may take weeks to heal.

It is the feeding polyps or gastrozooids which actually work on the prey. The last are the reproductive polyp or gonozooids. As the name suggests, they perform the function of reproduction.

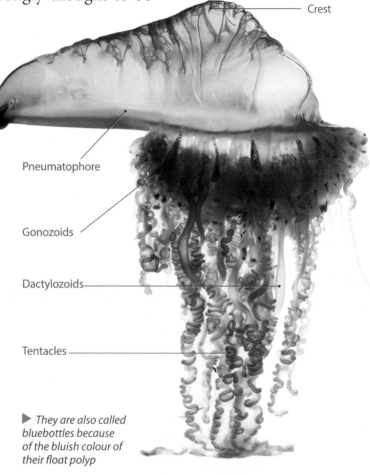

Crest

Pneumatophore

Gonozoids

Dactylozoids

Tentacles

▶ They are also called bluebottles because of the bluish colour of their float polyp

▶ A cluster of Portuguese man o' war, with the tops of their heads visible

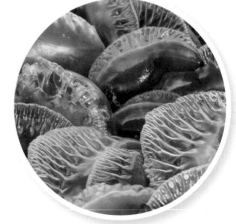

⊛ Incredible Individuals

Ever wonder where the names of different animals come from? William Elford Leach often named animals after people he knew. He named nine species in his lifetime, including several crustaceans. He named many species after an unknown woman named Caroline. He also named some after his friend John Cranch.

Soft-bodied Molluscs

Molluscs are highly adaptive soft-bodied invertebrate species from the phylum Mollusca. They are wholly or partially enclosed in a protective calcium carbonate shell secreted by the soft mantle which also covers their body. These are one of the most diverse groups in the animal kingdom alongside insects and vertebrates, with the possibility of 150,000 identified and unidentified species. There is immense ecological and structural variety in each group of molluscs.

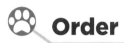

Order

Molluscs are classified into nine different groups, out of which two have been designated as extinct. These are wormlike organisms or Solenogastres; chitons or Polyplacophora; cap-shelled molluscs or Monoplacophora; slugs and snails or Gastropoda; hard-shelled organisms like clams or Bivalvia; tusk-shelled organisms or Scaphopoda; squid or Cephalopoda; Rostroconchia (extinct); and Helcionelloida (extinct).

Adaptability

Molluscs are proven to be highly adaptive as they have evolved into species that are present everywhere in nature, except air. Bivalves, gastropods, and cephalopods are usually seen in a marine environment but there are some species of gastropods that have successfully evolved and adapted themselves to land, with thousands of species existing terrestrially, taking advantage of sandy and muddy substrates to crawl, burrow, or to cement themselves to these surfaces.

Clams

Clams are found in shallow waters, in which they are protected by water currents and also because they have a cemented grip where they burrow or traverse over. They have shells that they open or close using their two adductor muscles. Certain species of Bivalvia clam have been discovered in the Pacific Ocean at a depth of more than 4,800 metres. The size of clams ranges from 0.1 millimetres in condylocardia to 1.2 metres in the giant clam of the Pacific and Indian Oceans.

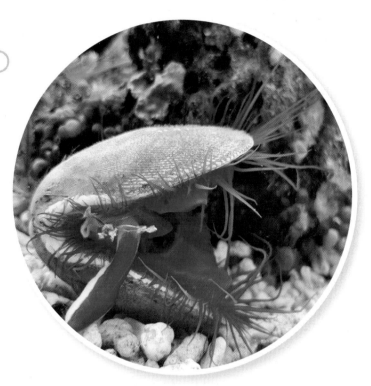

▲ *Shelled molluscs have powerful muscles called 'adductors', which help them shut the shell quickly to avoid predators*

Feeding and Survival

Clams draw in and expel water for the purpose of feeding and respiration through two separate tubes which are also called the siphons or 'neck'. This process helps accumulate food strained from the ongoing water currents, which is then transported to the mouth entangled in mucus. A few species of clams do not feed in the normal sense; they gain their nutrition from sulphur-oxidising bacteria that live symbiotically in the gill tissue. They are commonly found at marine hydrothermal vents and in sulphide-rich sediments.

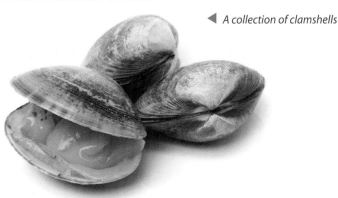

◀ *A collection of clamshells*

Isn't It Amazing!

Clams are an interesting and diverse species. A few clams, such as the gem clam, have internal fertilisation and development. There are clams or shell-based molluscs which produce the pearls we use as jewellery. Disco clams are known for putting on a show with reflected light.

Spectacular Tentacles

Octopuses are molluscs. They are called cephalopods, which means 'head-footed'. Unlike snails, in case of octopuses, their molluscan foot is located at the headend. The animal is named octopus because of the eight distinct arms of the invertebrate.

Facts of Physique

Octopuses have soft, round, sac-like bodies. They have large bulging eyes and a beak-like mouth hidden in the ring of arms. The powerful arms are covered with suction cups called suckers. These are used to catch prey, move over rocks, and swim.

An interesting fact about this invertebrate is that it has three hearts and nine brains. Two of its hearts supply blood to the gills, the breathing organ. The third heart is the organ heart, which supplies blood to the other organs.

Blue-blooded

The blood of an octopus is blue in colour because of the presence of hemocyanin, a copper-rich protein. This protein binds to the oxygen molecules, thus helping transport oxygen throughout the body.

▲ *Female octopus have to keep their eggs safe from predators as well as gently guide currents of water over them, so that they get a fresh supply of oxygen. They do this without leaving their side or eating. When the eggs hatch, the mother is so exhausted and starved, that she dies*

▲ *On mating, the female octopuses lay eggs on rocks. They are small, shaped like a teardrop and milky in appearance*

Intelligent Beings

Octopus brains are another story. One of them, the big one, controls the **nervous system**, while the remaining small brains control the animal's tentacles. Long ago, octopuses were thought to be dumb, but did you know they are one of the most intelligent invertebrates? They are known to recognise different colours, shapes, carry out simple tasks such as opening boxes, navigate through mazes, and solve simple problems.

Dwelling and Feeding

Octopuses are solitary creatures. They build dens with rocks that they move with their arms. Few do live near the water's surface, but most octopuses are deep-sea dwellers. They crawl on the ocean floors using their arms, looking for food to eat. They rise at dawn and dusk to look for food along the water's surface. Their favourite meals include crabs, shrimps, and lobsters.

Camouflage

Octopuses have pigment cells and special muscles which help them not just change colours but also match the texture and pattern of their surroundings. Sharks, dolphins and many other predators simply swim past such a camouflaged octopus.

Defence

If a camouflaged octopus is discovered, it squirts an ink-like liquid. This darkens the surrounding water, dulling the predator's sense of smell, giving the octopus enough time to escape. If this fails too and the octopus is caught by the predator by its arm, it just lets go the body part. Yes, it can regrow its arm! The beak-like mouth can also give a nasty bite to the predator and the saliva too is filled with venom.

Sticky Barnacles

If you own a ship, you might be familiar with barnacles. They are notorious for sticking to the bottom of a vessel, requiring the cleaner to use a lot of energy to get rid of them. Barnacles are crustaceans who live in the water.

🐾 Behaviour

Barnacles belong to the subclass Cirripedia. They live a sedentary life, which means that they stay in the same place for a long time. There are 850 species of marine barnacles and 260 species that act as parasites. They live in crustaceans like crabs.

Barnacles are covered with plates made of calcium carbonate. These are their **calcareous** plates. They choose different surfaces to stay on, but prefer places that are very active, such as an underwater volcano or the bottom of a ship, the bodies of whales and other larger animals, seaweed, rocks, and clams. They stick to these surfaces by releasing a fast-curing cement. It is such an efficient and sticky glue that researchers are trying to figure out how it can be used by humans.

🐾 Feeding Habits

Barnacles eat from their appendages. These are called cirri and look like little feathers. There is an opening on the barnacle from which the cirri reach out for food and retract. They eat microscopic organisms.

Many barnacles are circled by six calcareous plates and four more that behave like a door, opening and closing when the tide comes in and out. They close the door to conserve moisture and open it to look for food. Barnacles are also seen as a delicacy in some cultures. The Japanese use goose barnacles in their cooking, and so do the Spanish and Portuguese. Picoroco barnacle is used in Chile.

👤 In Real Life

Barnacles are **hermaphrodites.** It means that they possess both male and female reproductive organs. Some species might cross-fertilise while others fertilise themselves. Barnacles reproduce around six times a year. In cross-fertilisation, another barnacle might release sperm from a retractable tube that enters 6–8 inches into the partner's shell.

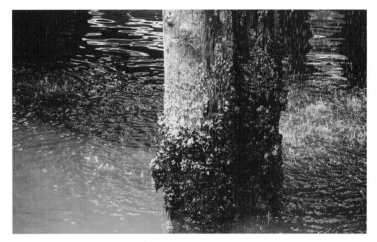

▲ Barnacles live for 8-20 years

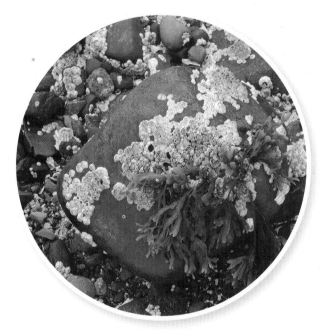

▲ Barnacles are free-floating, but eventually attach themselves to rocks, shell, or other objects

▼ The gooseneck barnacle resembles the fleshy stalk in the region of the goose's neck. This led ancient people to believe that the geese grew from the goose barnacle

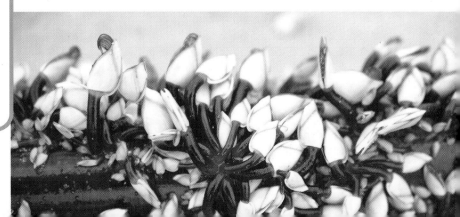

Floating Sea Otters

Not to be confused with otters, sea otters are marine animals. They are seen in the Pacific Ocean in North America and also in Asia. While they might spend their entire day in the water, some sleep on the shore. Their nostrils and ears have adapted to close when they are in water.

Otter Behaviour

Sea otters are often photographed floating on their backs on the surface of the water. They look like they are happily resting. Often, they float in a group or pair. They look for kelp forests and seaweed to use as an anchor in moving waters.

While they are floating, sea otters hold on their chests the rocks that they found ashore. They repeatedly hit the shellfish they have collected against the rocks to break them open and eat what is inside. They eat crabs, fish, octopuses, and sea urchins in the same way.

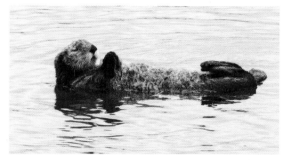

▲ Sea otters can remain submerged in water for over 5 minutes

On Their Backs

It seems as if sea otters do everything on their backs. They give birth in the water. Then, the mother otter cares for her young, while they are both on their backs. To feed their babies, they hold the infants against their chests. Sea otters learn to hunt for food and swim while they are still growing.

An adult sea otter grows to be 100–160 centimetres in length. It weighs 16–40 kilograms. They have slightly red or dark brown coats. These coats are valuable to human beings, so much so that sea otters almost went extinct because of how much they were hunted for their fur. While various countries made the effort to protect and conserve them, unfortunately, their numbers continue to decrease.

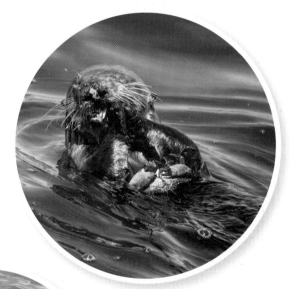

▲ A sea otter breaking apart a crab shell

◀ Sea otters have the thickest fur of any animal

▼ Sea otters hold their food with their hands and collect it on their stomachs as they float

Isn't It Amazing!

Sea otters always keep their fur clean. This is important as their fur repels water, keeping them dry and warm. Like human beings, they wash themselves after a meal. They rub the water into the coat using their paws and teeth.

The Whiskered Walruses

Walruses are mammals, but they are considered marine animals. This is because they spend most of their lives in or around the sea. Walruses are commonly seen near the Arctic Circle. They are accompanied by hundreds of their own kind.

Bodies

Walruses have bulky bodies with blubber. This blubber allows them to stay warm and comfortable in the harsh, cold Arctic climate. Walruses can slow their heartbeats to lower their temperatures when they are swimming in the cool waters.

Species

Walruses have two main species. One species is the Atlantic walrus that lives in the coastal regions of Greenland and Canada. The other species is the Pacific walrus that lives in Russia and Alaska. It migrates from the Bering Sea to the Chukchi Sea.

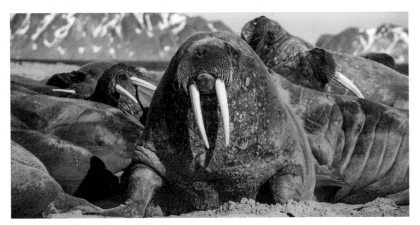

▲ Walruses can live up to 40 years

Tusks

Walruses have tusks and hair around their face that looks like a moustache. They use these tusks to lift themselves out of the cold Arctic waters. They seemingly walk using their tusks and use them to break small holes into the ice. These are called breathing holes. All walruses have tusks, regardless of their sex. They do not stop growing and even act as canine teeth. A regular tusk can grow up to 1 metre in length.

Whiskers

Walruses have sensitive whiskers. They use these whiskers to find food like clams and shellfish when they are swimming in the ocean. They might swim all the way down to a darker, deeper part of the ocean for food, at which time their whiskers are more important than their eyesight for navigation.

▼ A close-up shot of a walrus' tusks. Its whiskers are about as sensitive as a person's fingers

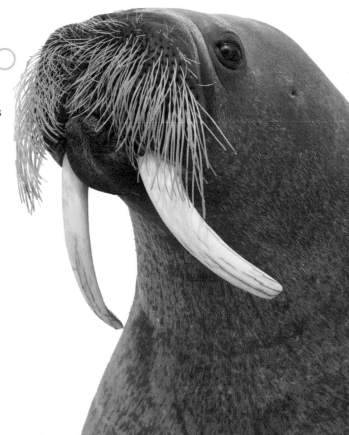

Walruses and Climate Change

As walruses live near icy regions, they are greatly affected by climate change. There is a big population of walruses in the Chukchi Sea of the Arctic Ocean. The ice in this sea has started melting and continues to melt at an alarming rate. As there is a change in the distribution of ice in the sea, the walruses' diet, movement, and mating habits are changing. Their population is slowly reducing. They are forced to change where they forage for food during autumn and summer.

In Real Life

In the past, the number of walruses was in decline due to hunting. They were hunted for their tusks, skin, meat, oil, and so on during the 18th and 19th centuries. They nearly faced extinction. After changes in laws, only certain local tribes are allowed to hunt for walruses.

Homely Habitats

Almost all organisms on this planet have homes. There are places that fish and amphibians inhabit because it suits their lifestyles the best. These habitats provide them with food, water, and shelter as per their needs. Let us take a look at some of these interesting places that are home for various marine animals, and some animals that make unique use of their environments.

🐾 Coral Reefs

Coral reefs are not only home to corals, but also to seahorses, clownfish, sea turtles, etc. Corals themselves are marine animals. They have small tentacle-like arms that allow them to eat food, such as plankton, from the water. Similar to the coral reefs are the kelp forests, another major home for marine animals. Sea lions, whales, and other marine animals eat the small critters that live in the leaves found in abundance here. On the other hand, marine animals like crabs and oysters live in estuaries.

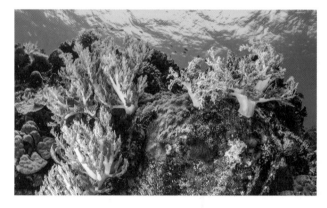

◀ *Each and every structure in the coral reef is alive and can die off*

🐾 Nile River

The Nile River is the longest in the world. It is home to more than 100 species of fish as well as amphibians. The smaller fish are often eaten by birds and bigger fish. The big fish, such as the Nile perch, are eaten by human beings.

The Nile perch can grow as long as 6.6 feet and weigh almost 200 kilograms. It is a predator which eats smaller cichlid fish. Also inhabiting the Nile River are the African lungfish found closer to Lake Victoria.

◀ *The Nile perch is used to produce fish oil, which is healthy for human beings*

Mudbanks

Lungfish, like the name suggests, have one or two lungs along with their gills. They evolved in the Devonian Period. They are found in Australia, South America and Africa, and live on mudbanks. The 'lung', which is nothing but a modified swim bladder, helps them survive when their home pools dry up or they get stranded on riverbanks. They burrow into mud and breathe air with their lung.

▶ Lungfish have actually evolved from 4-footed land animals

Antarctica

In spite of extreme weather conditions, wherein the area faces temperatures on the minus scale almost throughout the year, it does show a lot of biodiversity. Apart from penguins, seals, whales, and sharks, smaller fish live here as well. However, no amphibian can survive this harsh cold climate.

Antarctic toothfish is a species which inhabits the seas close to the continent. How does it survive the cold? The fish can produce anti-freeze proteins in its tissues and blood.

Another interesting species found in the Southern Ocean is the mackerel icefish. It too carries the anti-freeze protein as seen in most Antarctic fish. The icefish are white-blooded, meaning that they lack haemoglobin, the oxygen-carrying red pigment found in other fish. They have many adaptations in them, mainly in the cardiovascular system, which help compensate for the lack of haemoglobin.

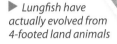

To Swim or To Walk

Mudskippers are small, tropical fish that show amphibious characteristics. They live in the swamps and estuaries of eastern Africa, and the Indian and Pacific Oceans.

Mudskippers are about 30 centimetres in length. Their strong pectoral fins help their movement on land. They prey on shrimps and other very small animals. When in water, they breathe with the help of gills, just like all fish do. But on land, they use special gill chambers that fill up with water. This keeps the gills moist and functional for several hours on land. Also, mudskippers can take in oxygen through their skin.

▲ Antarctic toothfish live to almost 50 years of age

◀ The mudskipper goes on land to fight, hunt for food, and even to mate

REPTILES & AMPHIBIANS

UNIQUE **CREATURES**

Amphibians and reptiles are related to each other. Reptiles actually evolved from amphibians. The ferocious crocodile, the slithering snake, the slow tortoise, and the colour-changing chameleon are all classified as reptiles. Even the mighty dinosaurs belong to the same group.

To understand reptiles, we need to go back in time—not just a few thousand years—but more than 300 million years, when a branch of **amphibians** evolved into reptiles.

But what are amphibians? The word 'amphibian' combines the Greek words for 'both' and 'life', denoting that these creatures live on land and in water. Most amphibians have lungs and also breathe through their skin. They need to keep their skin wet in order to absorb oxygen, so they secrete a type of mucous that keeps it moist.

◄ Frogs are amphibians as they spend parts of their lives on land and in water

▶ Although an alligator is a reptile, it can swim well in water and crawl on land

Evolution of Amphibians

The fossil record of amphibians has been poor until recently. However, new discoveries give us a clear picture of the history of amphibians. As the Silurian Period went on, the diverse species of fish continued to evolve. Scientists do not know for certain if they got tired of fighting off too many predators or if they had too much competition for food, but eventually some fish began to move towards land.

The Missing Pieces

The first animals to move to land and settle there were the arthropods. They had started their journey towards land 100 million years ago. The bodies of these animals were uniquely adapted to life on land as they had strong legs, light bodies, and hard **exoskeletons** that helped them conserve water.

These animals had to figure out how to conserve water, move, stay safe from predators, exchange gases (like oxygen and carbon dioxide), and learn to support themselves against the strong pull of gravity.

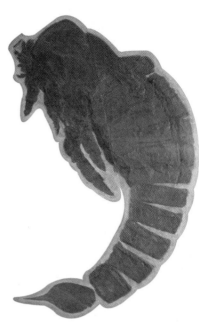

▲ *An extinct relative of the modern scorpion, called Slimonia, was one of the earliest animals to live on land along with mites and spiders*

The Story Begins

During the Devonian Period, land was occupied by arthropods and **tetrapods**. It is said the amphibians evolved from tetrapods and were related to the primitive **lobe-finned fish**. These fish probably had lungs that helped them breathe on land. Their bony limbs had digits at the ends that helped them crawl on land.

Eusthenopteron is a fossil belonging to the late Devonian Period. Scientists believe this animal was near the main line of

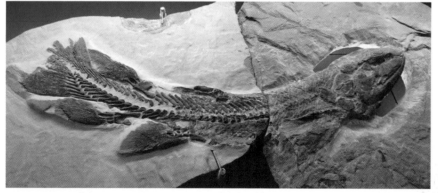

▲ *A beautifully preserved fossil of Eusthenopteron*

evolution from fish to amphibians. It was about six feet long, had a broad skull with teeth, and was a carnivore. The vertebral column was not well developed, but the fins had bony structures for support.

Eusthenopteron was not built for life on land. It probably lived in shallow waters, climbing small rocks and plants in search of food.

💡 Isn't It Amazing!

In the Late Triassic Period, amphibians reached gigantic proportions. There lived a giant salamander called *Metoposaurus algarvensis*. It was the size of a small car and perhaps even ate small dinosaurs!

▶ *An illustration of the Tiktaalik roseae*

Paving the Path

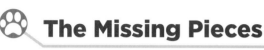

The fossil of an aquatic animal called *Tiktaalik roseae* was discovered in 2004 in Canada. It was a tetrapod and about nine feet long. It had sharp teeth and, unlike fish, it could move its head from side to side to look for prey and predators. It probably had arms with elbows, wrists, and shoulders. Hence, it is considered to be the first fish with limbs. It had a flat skull with bulging eyes like that of a modern crocodile, suggesting it swam beneath waters in lakes, streams, and swamps.

▶ *Ichthyostega were more advanced than Eusthenopteron and closer in relation to the first tetrapods*

Moving Towards Land

The fossil of *Ichthyostega*, an animal closely related to the tetrapods, was found in Greenland. It belonged to the late Devonian Period. The animal was about three feet in length. A unique feature of this animal was that each of its feet had seven toes. It did show aquatic traits such as a short snout, presence of a bone in the cheek region that covers the gills in fish, and small scales on the body. But, like tetrapods, it lacked gills, had bones supporting fleshy limbs, and strong ribs. *Ichthyostega* could leap and move on land.

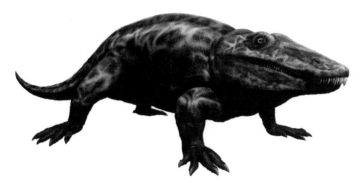

▲ *Being short with broad limbs might have helped the Eryops walk on land*

Landed

About 340 million years ago, the evolution of the first known family of amphibians took place. They were called the *temnospondyls*. *Eryops* is an example of this group. It had a stout body, large skull, and a strong vertebral column, suggesting the animal could move on land. Its teeth were sharp, indicating that it could have been a carnivore.

What Happened to Ancient Amphibians?

Ancient amphibians were one of the largest predators on land for millions of years. But in the Permian Period, about 280 million years ago, Earth's climate changed. This period marks the largest mass extinction in Earth's history. Wetlands and swamps were replaced by vast deserts. But amphibians needed water to reproduce and survive. The change in climate caused many of the amphibian species to die out.

Extinction and Resurgence

The Permian Mass Extinction was an event which wiped out more than 95 per cent of all life on Earth. This included the giant amphibian predators. However, a few survived in the shadows of the reptiles (dinosaurs).

During the Jurassic Period, the climate changed once again, giving rise to wetlands, and the surviving amphibians evolved to form the modern amphibians we know today, such as frogs, salamanders, and newts.

Incredible Individuals

Jodi Rowley is a biologist who studies amphibians, focusing on their diversity, environment and the threats to their existence. Today, it is said that one-third of all amphibian population is threatened with extinction and Jodi Rowley is taking measures for their conservation. She is mainly focussed on the conservation of Southeast Asian amphibians.

Characteristics of Amphibians

To us human beings, from where we stand at the highest position on the evolutionary scale, amphibians seem like just another set of animals that cohabit Earth with us. But these animals, which are at the base of the evolutionary scale, have many interesting tales to tell.

🐾 The Heart of the Matter

Fish and amphibians have similar structures for many internal organs such as the stomach, gall bladder, liver, and kidney. But their hearts are structured differently. A fish has a two-chambered heart, where one chamber receives blood and the other chamber pumps blood out.

On the other hand, amphibians have a three-chambered heart. The first chamber receives the oxygenated blood, the second chamber pumps it to the entire body, and the third chamber receives deoxygenated blood.

Amphibians hearts are like balloons where they can only take up a limited amount of gas. So, they diffuse the extra oxygen through their skin.

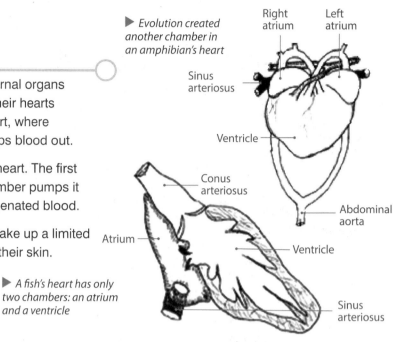

▶ *Evolution created another chamber in an amphibian's heart*

Right atrium

Left atrium

Sinus arteriosus

Ventricle

Conus arteriosus

Abdominal aorta

Atrium

Ventricle

Sinus arteriosus

▶ *A fish's heart has only two chambers: an atrium and a ventricle*

🐾 Spitting Frogs

Frogs can swallow insects whole by simply pushing their sticky tongues out. The saliva helps them capture the prey. To swallow the insect, a frog closes its eyes. This helps it push the insect down towards the throat. However, when a frog eats something poisonous, it simply spits out the contents of its stomach.

Yes, you read that right, the food in a frog's stomach can come out entirely through its mouth to discard the disagreeable contents. When a frog eats bombardier beetles, the insect might squirt boiling chemicals into the frog's stomach as a defence, so the frog will spit it out.

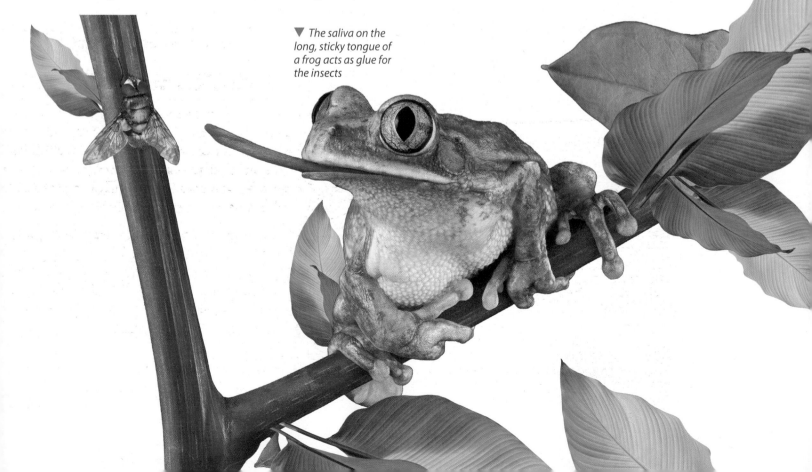

▼ *The saliva on the long, sticky tongue of a frog acts as glue for the insects*

The Blind Dragon

The olm is a blind salamander that lives in caves. It resorts to its other sensory organs to hunt for food. It has pale pink skin. It does not grow, instead it maintains its red feathery gills that form when it is a **larva**, even after it reaches maturity. It was once called a baby dragon because of the small size of its snake-like body. Olm salamanders can live for more than a hundred years.

The olm salamanders have existed for nearly 20 million years in the caves of Croatia and Slovenia, but chemical pollutants are now threatening the ancient animal's existence.

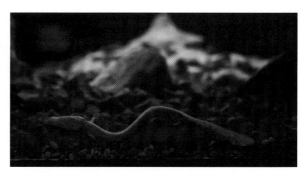

▲ *Olm salamanders eat crabs, snails and small insects*

Most Moist

Amphibians have a moist, slimy skin as seen in most frogs. This is one of the reasons amphibians stay near water. Few amphibians live in hostile environs, such as the African bullfrogs who endure the hot, harsh climate of southern Africa. They have skins with long ridges to prevent moisture loss.

Commonly seen in amphibians is the process of metamorphosis. As the immature larva develops, it undergoes bodily changes that make it distinct from the adult it grows into. For example, most amphibians spend the early years of their lives in water, but as adults they take to land.

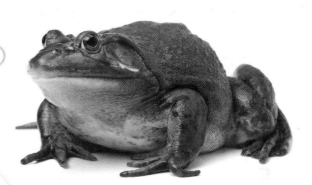

▲ *Have you ever seen a frog look dry? They always have slimy and moist skin as they need to stay moist for survival*

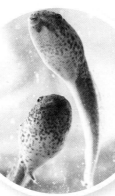

◄ *A close-up of the larva that frogs develop from*

To Catch a Fly

Research shows that frogs might have special spit that helps them catch flies. Their saliva is sticky, so frogs can extend their tongues and hold onto the flies that they catch. Their saliva, which is normally thick, liquefies to spread over the insect's body and then thickens again, effectively trapping it.

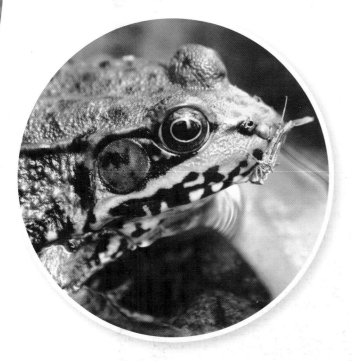

▲ *Once the insect is in their mouth, frogs use their eyeballs to swallow it. The eyeballs move to the mouth cavity and push down the food, exerting force that liquifies the saliva and releases the insect*

⊚ Incredible Individuals

In the 17th century, a woman named Catharina Geisslerin in Germany claimed that she had swallowed tadpoles from a swamp. She claimed that these tadpoles were happily living in her body as frogs. She also claimed that drinking milk caused these frogs to jump out of her mouth. Surprisingly, she managed to duplicitously convince physicians that this was true by vomiting frogs in front of them.

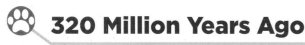

Evolution of Reptiles

The reptiles that we see on Earth today can be traced back to small lizards. These lizards roamed the planet more than 350 million years ago. They laid amniotic eggs which allowed them to move from water to land. Slowly, these land vertebrates grew in size.

🐾 320 Million Years Ago

The reptiles separated into two groups—**synapsids** and **sauropsids**. Synapsids were the early ancestors of modern mammals. Sauropsids evolved into modern birds, reptiles and dinosaurs. Though both were vertebrates, for a few million years, the synapsids became the dominant species. *Hylonomus* and *Paleothyris* were the earliest reptiles.

▲ *Hylonomus were small, preferred to live in swamps and fed on insects*

🐾 245 Million Years Ago

The Permian Mass Extinction occurred over 252 million years ago and lasted for nearly 15 million years. It wiped out 95 per cent of marine animals and 70 per cent of land animals, including most synapsids. However, the sauropsids survived and even thrived while the synapsids declined in number. This came to be known as the **Triassic takeover**.

🐾 The Mesozoic Era

Large dinosaurs gradually evolved from sauropsids nearly 225 million years ago. They dominated the land and became one of the most important groups of animals of the **Mesozoic Era**. This era was divided into the Triassic Period, the Jurassic Period, and the Cretaceous Period.

During the Triassic Period, both dinosaurs and reptiles evolved rapidly, but it is only during the Jurassic Period that the diversity of the dinosaur species evolved. Many dinosaurs became extinct towards the end of the Mesozoic Era, but the reptiles survived.

🐾 230 Million Years Ago

Evolving from their small lizard-like ancestors, reptiles began to rule not only on land but also in air. The major predators of this time were the Archosaurs. They were ancestors of the present-day crocodiles but were very different in appearance. Most animals belonging to this species had strong forelimbs and long hind legs. They had two skull openings, one in the snout and another in the lower jaw. But the function of these openings is unknown.

▼ *Proterosuchus was the first template for the modern crocodile. It had a slight downward curve in the upper jaw*

▶ *Archosaur means the 'ruling reptile'. They were divided into the Pseudosuchia (crocodiles) and the Ornithosuchia (birds)*

The Flying Reptiles

Pterosaurs, or 'flying reptiles', ruled the skies for about 150 million years. They should not be confused with dinosaurs, but they did belong to the group of archosaurs. They had no competition till the birds arrived millions of years later, as they were the first flying vertebrates.

Pterosaurs had light, hollow bones and their wing surface was formed by a membrane of skin similar to that of the modern bats. This membrane stretched across their thin fingers. Another membrane stretched from the wrist to their shoulder. This allowed them to fly with ease. They had small, sharp needle-like teeth in their jaws with which they could catch fish while still in flight.

▲ *Archelons were about 12 feet in length*

▲ *Some scientists believe pterosaurs walked on their hind legs, while others believe they walked on all fours with their wings folded by their sides*

▼ *Sarcosuchus fossils show that the gigantic animal might have spanned 10–12 metres and weighed around 8 metric tons*

Dominating the Seas

In the oceans, marine reptiles had become the dominant species. The long-necked Elasmosaurus was one of the largest sea creatures that had needle-like teeth perfectly suited for catching fast-moving fish. The first turtles evolved during the Cretaceous Period. The Late Cretaceous Period had turtles called Archelons. They protected themselves from predators with shells that were similar to those of the modern sea turtles. They moved in the water by pushing themselves forward with their front feet. Archelon died out with the dinosaurs around 65 million years ago.

Evolution Continues

Crocodiles and lizards continued to survive and evolve alongside dinosaurs. The crocodiles grew to extremely large sizes, such as the Sarcosuchus which preyed on some species of dinosaurs. These monstrous crocodiles died out with the dinosaurs.

Some lizards lost their legs and became the first snakes. These snakes were mostly constrictors, like the modern pythons, but smaller. At some point during the evolution process, the 'Sonic hedgehog' gene switched off in snakes. This gene is necessary for the growth of limbs, and gets its name from the spines that grow from the embryo during the limb-development stage. So, snakes became limbless reptiles. However, a genetic mutation could cause them to grow limbs once again.

◀ *While most were small, the Titanoboa is the largest known member of the serpent family. They lived near the end of the Cretaceous Period, and weighed around 1,135 kilograms, and had a length of roughly 13 metres!*

Reptilian Features

The word 'reptile' refers to the animals' creeping and crawling movement. Reptiles are vertebrates, which means they have backbones which support and give shape to their bodies. They live in hot deserts, swamps, oceans, and forests. Animals can only be classified as reptiles if they possess certain characteristic features.

Cold-blooded

Reptiles are ectothermic or cold-blooded animals. Like amphibians and fish, reptiles cannot regulate their body temperature. They need sunlight and shade too. That is why, in their natural habitats, chameleons have been observed basking on hillside rocks in winters. Since they are cold-blooded, reptiles cannot survive without heat.

They lie perpendicular to the Sun, so that they can absorb a lot of sunlight. If it gets too hot, the reptile will lie parallel to the Sun or look for a shady spot. A chameleon will lighten the colour of its skin if it gets too hot, a crocodile might keep its mouth wide open, while a snake might burrow into the soil.

Reptiles in the desert region, such as Gila monsters, are nocturnal in summers because their bodies cannot handle the harsh heat during the day. However, if the temperature is tolerable, they can be diurnal.

Tough Skin

Having tough, scaly skin is the key to survival in reptiles. The skin not only acts as a protective covering, but also prevents loss of water, which saves it from drying up. The scales are made of keratin, the structural protein present in the hair and fingernails of human beings. The scales may be tiny—as found in dwarf geckos, or large—as seen in lizards. Even turtles have scales called scutes, which are arranged in a staggered manner. The scales on a crocodile are called armour.

Incredible Individuals

Back in 1992, Steve Irwin filmed a documentary with his wife, Terri Raines, called *The Crocodile Hunter*. It became so popular that he was given the opportunity to film more of the documentary, of which currently there are 50 episodes. 'Crocodile Hunter' became his nickname, even though he never actually hunted a crocodile. In fact, he was known for his close encounters with dangerous animals and his work with conservationists to help save the crocodiles.

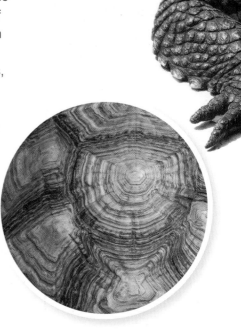

▶ A turtle's shell has scutes made up of keratin. Though they act as the shell, they are built like a nail, beak, or horn

Eggs

Most reptiles lay eggs. Without the special feature of the amniotic eggs, reptiles could never have moved onto land. These types of eggs have leathery or hard shells which protect the embryo. The eggshell allows the flow of air but prevents vital fluids from leaking out. Inside the eggs, there are a series of fluid-filled membranes which help the embryo survive and develop.

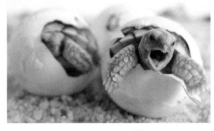

▲ *Like most creatures that are born in eggs, turtles also have egg teeth. They help the baby creature to break out of its shell*

Eyes

Reptiles are dependent on their sharp vision to catch prey. Crocodiles have eyes specially adapted for hunting at night, while chameleons can move their eyes independent of each other. This helps them scan their surroundings for extremely tiny insects. However, snakes such as pythons and rattlesnakes have poor eyesight. They use what is called 'heat vision', which helps snakes sense the heat given off by warm-blooded creatures, through small openings in front of their eyes.

▼ *Crocodilians and birds are the only surviving dinosaurians*

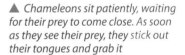

▲ *Chameleons sit patiently, waiting for their prey to come close. As soon as they see their prey, they stick out their tongues and grab it*

Teeth

Reptiles have no specialised teeth such as canines, incisors or molars, like mammals do. They have a long row of conical teeth to catch and chew the prey, as seen in crocodiles and alligators. These animals either swallow the prey whole or cut it into bite-size portions before swallowing. Turtles have sharp edges on their jaws, which they use to bite off seaweed and other foods. Snakes have fangs. The number, placement and shape of teeth varies among reptiles.

In Real Life

The incubation temperature among crocodiles and some turtles, at a certain stage of development, determines the sex of the embryo. For example, in red-eared slider turtles, if eggs are incubated below 28° C, the hatchlings will be male. If the temperature is above 31° C, the hatchlings will be female, and in the temperatures between, it could be either male or female.

Orderly Amphibians

The amphibian world is made up of many orders. All are extinct, except three surviving orders, namely Gymnophiona, Anura, and Caudata.

Order Gymnophiona

It is also called order Apoda, which refers to limbless animals. Its members are known as caecilians. There are 206 known species of smooth-skinned, limbless, worm-like, burrowing amphibians in this order.

Caecilians live in humid, tropical regions around the world. They hunt using the two tentacles located near their mouths that help them sense the environment. Terrestrial caecilians eat soft-bodied creatures like earthworms, while the aquatic caecilians feed on eels, fish, and invertebrates.

▲ The name 'caecilians' is derived from the Latin word 'caecus' which means 'blind'

▼ Frogs are commonly brown, green or grey with very few colourful species

In Real Life

Ichthyophis beddomei or Beddome's caecilian is a yellow-striped worm-like amphibian found in the Western Ghats of India. It is a freshwater animal, living comfortably in the soil and in the tropical evergreen forests. It is also found in the agricultural areas of this region. If disturbed, it produces a whitish fluid and disappears into the soil.

Order Anura

It is also called order Salientia and it consists of around 6,623 species of amphibians. Members of this group have short, broad bodies with no neck and tail. They have long powerful hindlimbs for leaping, webbed feet for swimming, and long, sticky tongues to catch insects. They have well-developed eyelids. Frogs and toads belong to this group.

Order Caudata

Order Caudata is also called order Urodela and it consists of 740 species of amphibians. This group of amphibians have distinct heads, trunks and tails. They have weak limbs, smooth skin, and teeth present on both jaws. Newts and salamanders belong to this group.

▼ Caudata means 'tail-bearing', and predictably, the species that belong to this order have tails

Outstanding Amphibians

The *Paedophryne amauensis* holds the record of being the world's smallest known frog. As big as a housefly, it is said to be about 7.7 millimetres in length. It inhabits the rainforest floor of New Guinea but is very difficult to spot due to its size.

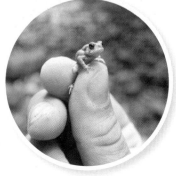

► Scientists believe that these frogs evolved to be tiny so that they could feed on little invertebrates for survival

The Class Reptilia

There are more than 10,000 species classified as reptiles. They are found in all continents except Antarctica. Scientists have further divided this class of animals into four orders, with each order having features special to that particular group; for example crocodiles are the only reptiles with a four-chambered heart.

The Four Orders

The four reptile orders are Testudinata—consisting of turtles, Crocodilia—consisting of crocodiles and alligators, Rhynchocephalia—consisting of tuataras, and Squamata—consisting of snakes and lizards.

01 Order: Testudinata

Characteristics: Bony shells cover most of these reptiles' bodies. They have rounded backs, flat bellies, no teeth and sharp jaws (for cutting food). They are egg-laying reptiles.
Habitat: They live in saltwater, freshwater, and semi-arid regions.
Examples: Musk turtles, mud turtles, and Hermann's tortoise

▲ *A tortoise*

02 Order: Crocodilia

Characteristics: These reptiles have sharp vision and big snouts. They use their powerful tails to swim, keeping their eyes and nostrils above the water.
Habitat: They are found in streams, lakes, rivers, and swamps.
Examples: Gharials, Nile crocodiles, and Caimans

▲ *A crocodile*

03 Order: Rhynchocephalia

Characteristics: Belonging to a sister group of order Squamata. There is only one surviving species called tuataras. This reptile has rows of spines running along the back of the neck and backbone. Their young display the remnants of a third eye, but this gradually gets covered by scales within a few months.
Habitat: They live in the islands off the coast of New Zealand.

04 Order: Squamata

a. (Suborder: Serpentes or Snakes)

Characteristics: These reptiles have long and slender bodies. They usually lack legs but have broad scales on the belly to allow forward movement. They do not have eyelids and ears.
Habitat: They are found in all environments where reptiles are found such as forests, mountains, and deserts.
Examples: Rattle snakes, anacondas, king cobras, and coral snakes

▲ *A cobra*

▼ *A garden lizard*

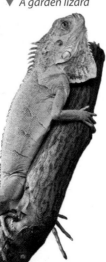

b. (Suborder: Lacertilia or Lizards)

Characteristics: Most reptiles belonging to this suborder have four legs and a tail. They have eyelids and openings for the ears. Many lay eggs, but some give birth to the young ones.
Habitat: They are found in all environments where reptiles are found such as forests, mountains, and deserts.
Examples: Geckos, komodo dragons, iguanas, and monitor lizards

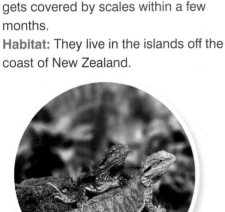

▲ *It takes 9 months for tuataras to lay eggs, which then take 13 months to hatch!*

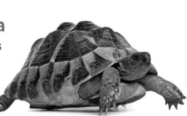

Newts and Salamanders

Newts and salamanders—the words often go together. But are they the same thing?
A newt is always a salamander, but not all salamanders are newts. The salamanders that
live on land are called newts. Salamanders are reptiles that retain their tails even after
they grow into adults. A salamander looks a little like a frog and a little like a lizard.

🐾 Mudpuppy

The mudpuppy is a salamander that is mistakenly believed to be capable
of barking, hence it is also called a waterdog. This salamander has external,
red gills which it grows at the larval stage and never loses, even after
becoming an adult.

Mudpuppies spend their entire lives in water as they have no lungs. They
live at the bottom of pools, rivers, streams, and lakes. When water dries up
where they live, especially during summers, they burrow in mud until their
pools fill up again.

Mudpuppies are found in abundance in the USA and parts of Canada.
They hide in vegetation or behind logs and rocks, emerging at night to eat
crayfish, snails, and worms. Unlike in many other species, females guard
their eggs until they are hatched.

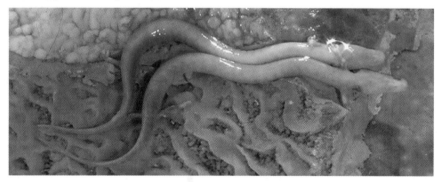

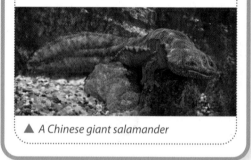
◄ *A diminishing mudpuppy population can be a
symptom of environmental problems in an area,
as the animal is sensitive to pollutants*

🐾 Kaiser's Spotted Newt

Kaiser's spotted newt is a small newt. It grows to a length of 10 or
14 centimetres as an adult. It has a black or white body dotted with
stripes, and spots that are orange or red in colour. It is impossible
to tell the male and female of the species apart when they are seen
outside of the breeding season. During the breeding season, the
male has a visibly rounded and enlarged cloacal region, while the
female has a volcano-shaped cloacal region.

While most salamanders live in caves, the Kaiser's spotted newt lives
in the Zagros Mountains in Iran. This is why it is also called the Iranian
harlequin newt. This is surprising for a newt as most salamanders like
shady and humid spots. Instead, the Kaiser's spotted newt lives in a
region where water is only available for three or four months. During
this period, the Kaiser's spotted newt eats a lot and finds a mate.
Then, it goes underground and rests in the soil. It breathes slowly,
has a low heart rate, and barely eats until water is available again.

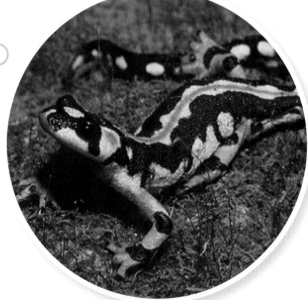

▲ *Salamanders look for moist and cool places
to live in*

A Tad of a Journey

Imagine an army of red-eyed tree frogs coming your way. An 'army' is what a group of red-eyed tree frogs is called. But you would only get to see the red-eyed tree frogs in person in Central America and Mexico. It inhabits tropical rainforests and likes to live near ponds and rivers.

 ## The Egg Stage

During the monsoon season, the females lay a lot of eggs on the underside of a leaf, just above a pond or a river. They might also lay the eggs in water.

The females choose the spot carefully, as the eggs need to be moist all the time. Once they lay the eggs, the males fertilise them.

The eggs of frogs do not have hard, protective shells like reptile eggs. In fact, eggs laid by frogs are quite weak in comparison. They need to be covered with water, otherwise they dry up and die. The eggs absorb the water around them and become much bigger.

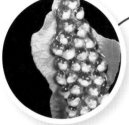

▲ *Eggs laid by red-eyed tree frog*

 ## Hatched Eggs

After six days, when the eggs are ready to hatch, the tadpoles energetically swim around inside the egg. This energetic movement breaks the egg and releases the tadpoles. The moisture from the hatched eggs pushes the tadpoles into the pond water beneath.

The red-eyed tree frogs lay eggs that decide to hatch after carefully assessing the vibrations or signals that they pick up from their surroundings.

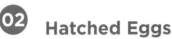 ## Tadpole Stage

After hatching, the embryonic tadpoles enter a new phase of their lives. They might be able to live outside water for 20 hours, but they need to move to the water to feed on algae. They breathe with their gills and swim using their tails. Within a week, they start to develop lungs and slowly lose their tails. This marks the beginning of the metamorphosis stage of their growth cycle.

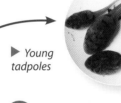

▶ *Young tadpoles*

▲ *The tadpole stage of a frog*

04 Metamorphosis

During this stage, the tadpoles begin to change into small brown froglets. This next phase is about the tadpoles developing legs. The tadpoles develop hind legs first. During this stage, the frog's head becomes distinct and the body elongates. The growth is aided by a diet of insects.

▲ *Metamorphosis of the tadpole*

▲ *The tail is now elongated and the tadpole has visible legs*

 ## Young Adult Stage

This stage comes two or three months after birth. The tadpole is now a tiny brown froglet. Barring a tiny stub for a tail, the frog looks like an adult. At this stage, the tail is being rapidly absorbed into the body. The frog leaves the water and moves onto trees. It can survive in both water and land like all amphibians.

▼ *The green colour of the frog acts as a camouflage when it sits on leaves*

06 Adult Stage

In the next few weeks, the frog turns green in colour. It develops blue and yellow stripes on its sides, orange feet, bluish thighs and the signature bright red eyes. It is now an adult, capable of taking care of itself and fighting its predators.

Frogs and Toads

There are around 7,411 species of frogs and toads in the world. They are found all over the world, except in Antarctica. However, they prefer warmer climatic conditions; hence, there is a greater population in the tropics. Of these, the reticulated glass frogs are especially interesting.

🐾 Reticulated Glass Frog

The reticulated glass frog is tiny—about the size of a coin—with see-through skin on its underside. If you ever get a view of the frog from underneath, you would be able to see its insides including its beating heart! The upper side is light green with spots.

The frog is found in the rainforests of Ecuador, Panama, Costa Rica, and Colombia. It eats the plants that grow along the streams in these forests. It is a nocturnal amphibian that cleverly uses its see-through underside to blend into the leaves to hide from dangerous predators.

▶ *To this day, scientists cannot confirm the reason for the frog having such see-through skin on the underside of its body*

🐾 Rough Males

The males of this species guard their territories fiercely. They repeatedly squeak at their predators or even other frogs who might try to trespass. If the squeaks do not scare them away, the male reticulated glass frogs wrestle them into leaving. On the other hand, if the red-eyed tree frog wants to escape a predator, it reveals its bright orange legs from underneath and bulges out its bright red eyes, shocking the predator momentarily. This gives the red-eyed tree frog a chance to escape quickly.

🐾 Colourful Leaps

Red-eyed tree frogs have suction-cup toes which help them attach to the underside of the leaves where they rest during daytime. At night, these frogs feed on crickets, moths, grasshoppers, and smaller frogs. Interestingly, unlike many other frog species which lay eggs directly in the water, the red-eyed tree frog lays them on a leaf.

▼ *Reticulated glass frogs are carnivorous and feed on different kinds of insects for survival*

▶ *Red-eyed tree frogs have small tadpoles that need to feed on insects to survive and grow. They grow into brown froglets, and only turn green as adults*

Responsible Fathers

Red-eyed tree frog females lay eggs on the underside of the leaves. The bunch of eggs they lay at once is called a 'clutch' and these eggs stick on the leaves because of a jelly-like substance.

Then, the males guard the eggs until they are hatched. They protect the eggs from wasps who might come to eat the eggs. The spotted green upper side of the frog resembles the cluster of eggs it is trying to protect. This camouflage pattern confuses the predator trying to get close to the actual eggs. These frogs have even been known to kick away predatory wasps.

In Real Life

If you kiss a common frog, no prince will appear, as it did in the fairy-tale *The Frog Prince*. Instead, you will get a slimy feel and a bad infection because frogs are known to carry bacteria called 'Salmonella'. Never try touching a wild frog or a toad; you never know what toxins they might carry!

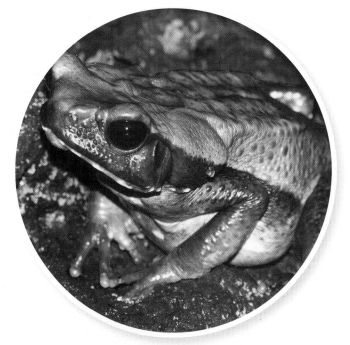

▲ *Smooth-sided toads are relatively sooth compared to the thicker, bumpier, and dry skins of most toads*

Smooth-sided Toad

Smooth-sided toads are medium-sized animals. The skin of the toad is spotted and brown. This acts as a camouflage, making it easy for the toad to hide on the forest floor. The smooth appearance is deceptive, as the warty skin with toxin glands is present in these toads as well, it is just not as obvious.

The smooth-sided toad has warts behind its eyes called the parotid glands. These produce dangerous toxins which can interfere with the predator's heart, even leading to death sometimes.

It is seen in the rainforests of countries such as Brazil, Colombia, Guyana, Ecuador, Suriname, and Venezuela. The animal can remain active all through the day and night and eats mostly insects.

Sign of Warning

An oriental fire-bellied toad looks like a regular toad with black spots covering its green skin. It blends well with the leaves and trees found in its habitats located in China, Korea, parts of Japan, and southern Russia.

The toad has a secret weapon; its skin secretes toxins. When it feels threatened, it rolls on its back and reveals its black and red underside, as it wants to warn the predator about the effects of eating it. In other words, it tries to tell the predator to stay away or it might die due to poisoning.

▼ *The oriental fire-bellied toad lives in ponds and streams*

Incredible Individuals

A herpetologist is a person who studies amphibians and reptiles. Ross Allen was a famous herpetologist, born in the USA. He developed anti-venoms after studying snakes. He also handled the animals used in movies such as *Tarzan Finds a Son*.

Turtle or Tortoise?

Are you confused about which is which? All tortoises are turtles, but not all turtles are tortoises! To make it simpler, 'turtle' is the broad name used for any animal which belongs to order Testudinata. Apart from a few structural differences between turtles and tortoises, the easiest way to differentiate between the two is the habitat that they are adapted to. Tortoises aren't adapted to water.

The Turtle Checklist

You know it is a turtle if:

✔ It lives in water. Some turtles live in freshwater, some in saltwater and some are amphibious, that is, they live both on land and in water;

✔ It is an omnivore, eating both plants and animals;

✔ It has a flattened and streamlined dome, allowing it to easily swim in water;

✔ It is aquatic or amphibious. Turtles have webbed feet which aid swimming. It is only the sea turtles which have proper flippers, which they use to swim long distances in the ocean.

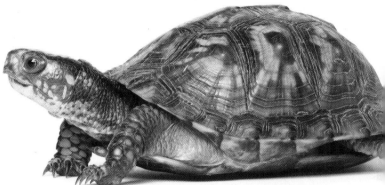

▲ Unlike most turtles, the Eastern box turtle has a dome-shaped shell

The Tortoise Checklist

You know it is a tortoise if:

✔ It is a terrestrial animal;

✔ It eats plants; though, there are a few varieties living in humid forest regions which are known to consume flesh and other insects;

✔ It has a large, high, dome-like shell. Unless it is the pancake tortoise that lives in Kenya, Tanzania and Zimbabwe. The pancake tortoise has a softer, more flat shell which helps it squeeze between rocks;

✔ It has stalky hind legs like an elephant's, designed to aid walking on land.

▲ A sea turtle gliding through water using its flippers

▲ Gopher tortoises use their legs to make burrows as deep as 10 feet into the ground

Isn't It Amazing!

The turtle is considered to be a sign of good luck in many cultures across the world. In India, the tortoise or 'kurma' in Sanskrit, is supposed to be the second incarnation of Lord Vishnu. Ancient Egyptians wore amulets depicting turtles as they believed this would keep them healthy. Turtles were also considered as the enemy of Ra, or Re, who was the Sun God.

Story of the Neck

Turtles are divided into two groups depending on how they tuck their necks inside their shells. The hidden-necked turtles can hide their heads completely inside their shells, while the side-necked turtles can turn their heads to one side and hide them just under the edge of their shells. Turtles or tortoises usually hide their heads for protection against any threats in the environment.

◀ The matamata turtle from South America can turn its head to one side

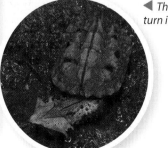

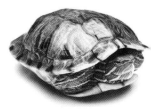

◀ A mud turtle with its head hidden inside its shell

Alike but Unlike

Can you tell a crocodile and an alligator apart? How about a worm lizard and a small snake? Scientists might have divided reptiles into orders, species and even families in bigger classifications, but there are a few animals which look so similar that it is difficult to make out who's who. So, let's learn to differentiate between these species.

🐾 Cousins

Alligators and crocodiles belong to order Crocodilia. So, if you want to refer to them as a group, you say 'crocodilians' but the word 'crocodile' isn't as inclusive.

Both are large, toothy predators, with long snouts, armours on their backs, and powerful tails. At a glance, they look so alike that it is hard to tell the difference between them. But here is how they are different from each other:

- Alligators have a wide head with the snout rounded into a U-shape, while crocodiles have narrow heads with snouts ending in sharp V-shapes.

- Both have one large tooth on the lower jaw. In the case of alligators, the tooth fits into a pit of the upper jaw and is not visible when the mouth is shut. However, in crocodiles, the tooth fits into a notch in the upper jaw but is still visible when the mouth is shut.

- Alligators are usually grey or black, while crocodiles are mostly olive or a pale brown in colour.

- Alligators prefer to live in freshwater, while crocodiles tend to be comfortable in saltwater.

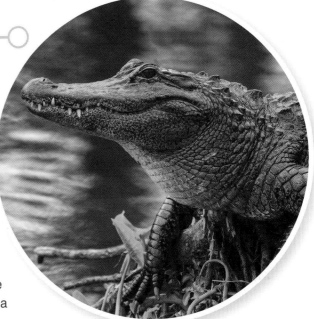

▲ *An American alligator, also called the Alligator mississipiensis, at the edge of a freshwater lake*

👤✓ In Real Life

There are only two species in the genus Alligator—the American alligator, which is found throughout the southeastern coast of the USA, and the critically endangered Chinese alligator that lives in the Anhui province of China.

▶ *The Nile crocodile, Africa's largest crocodile, is a menacing maneater*

Crawling Crocodilians

While on the one hand crocodilians are ruthless killers, they also fiercely guard their young ones. They live by the riverbanks and are among the most endangered species in the world. Their dwindling numbers are a result of global warming and human activity.

Gharials

Also called gavials, they have long, thin snouts and are mainly found in Asia. Their numbers are so low that the gharial has been declared as a critically endangered species by the International Union of Conservation of Nature (IUCN).

A Vanishing Home

Once upon a time, this reptile was found in abundance in countries like India, Pakistan, Nepal, and Myanmar. Today, it can only be found in India along the Son, Chambal, and Girwa rivers; and in Nepal, along the Narayani River.

What caused this decline? Around 98 per cent of the gharial population was lost to hunting for use in traditional medicine. Also, human beings have changed the courses of rivers to suit their needs. This has dried up many riverbeds, which were home to these precious reptiles.

A Pot for a Name

The males of these species have a bulb-like growth on their long snout, which resembles a *'ghara'*, which in Hindi means 'pot'; that is why this reptile is called 'gharial'. Males use these bulbous growths to call out and blow bubbles during the mating season to attract mates.

▼ *Not only are gharials critically endangered, but their population is also declining*

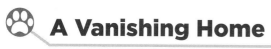

What Do They Look Like?

An adult gharial is close to almost 907 kilograms and can be 12–15 feet in length. Males are usually larger than females. These reptiles have weak legs and adults are unable to raise their bodies once on land. The long snout has sensory cells which detect vibrations created in water. The reptile, on sensing these vibrations, moves its head from side to side with force and tracks down the prey. It then grabs it firmly in its jaw, which has more than a hundred teeth. Adults mostly eat fish; however, young gharials are seen eating invertebrates found in the waters.

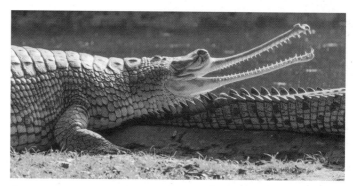

▲ *A giant gharial with a long snout*

The Creation

Gharials usually mate in the dry season. The female lays eggs near slow-moving water around the riverbank, where she digs a hole to lay eggs. Unlike many other reptiles, she does not leave the nest unguarded.
The eggs hatch in about 70 days and the hatchlings stay with their mother for weeks or even months, until they are ready to survive on their own.

We Are Crocodilians Too

Caimans are several species of reptiles belonging to the Crocodilian family. They are found in Central and South America. These are carnivores, living along the riverbanks or any other type of water bodies such as ponds or lakes. Like others in the order, they lay eggs, build nests and guard their young ones.

The spectacled caiman, as the name suggests, has a bony ridge between its eyes that looks like the nosepiece of an eyeglass. This reptile has made its home in an area between southern Mexico and Brazil.

▼ *Caimans are also called caymans. They were once sold to people as pets*

◀ *At night, when light is shown on them, the spectacled caiman's eyes reflect red light, making it easy to spot them in the dark*

The Yacare caiman is found in central parts of South America. It loves to feast on piranhas. About three decades ago, it was at the brink of extinction, thanks to armed gangs which killed them for their skin. The Brazilian government banned poaching, raising their numbers to almost ten million today.

Talking Eggs

Did you know crocodile eggs can get noisy just before hatching? When the babies are fully grown inside the egg, they call out to their siblings, telling them it is time to hatch; and to their mother, asking her to uncover the nest.

The Loving Crocodiles

They might be ferocious otherwise, but female crocodiles are gentle, caring mothers. Not only do they care for the eggs, but when they hatch, the mothers carry the newborn in their jaws into the water. If the mother hears a call of distress from her child, she rushes to the rescue. She also calls out to them when she wants them to assemble around her.

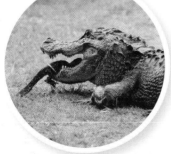

▶ *The mother crocodile does not shut her jaw, because it might hurt her babies*

▶ *Crocodiles lay 10–60 eggs at a time*

Stealthy Hunters

All crocodilians have a knack for hunting. They lurk underwater, with just their eyes and nostrils peeping above the surface. They can be as still as a log for hours together. Relying on their excellent eyesight, the moment they spot a prey, they swim over and catch it in their jaws in a matter of seconds.

👤 In Real Life

Crocodiles, alligators, caimans, and gharials are famous for their precious skin which is converted to bags, belts, and other items. Crocodile meat is also considered to be a delicacy in parts of the world. Most countries have banned the killing of these animals in the wild, yet poachers lurk as the skin and meat get a huge price in international markets.

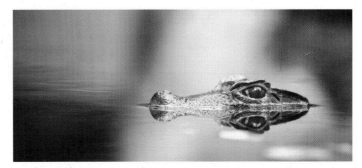

▲ *A caiman hiding underwater*

The World of Snakes

You know a snake when you see it. The animal is covered with overlapping scales. Larger ones protect the reptile's belly. These horizontally arranged scales enhance the snake's ability to slide on the ground or climb up a tree. Snakes shed their outer layer of skin in a process called **moulting**. The colours and patterns of snakeskin vary from one species to another.

The Mouth

Did you know a snake's mouth can open really wide? They have a special jaw that allows them to swallow whole a prey much larger than their size. It is the forked tongue of the snake which picks up the smell. It picks up chemical molecules from the surroundings and sends information to a special organ called Jacobson's organ, situated in the head. Here, the information is processed, and it helps the snake track down its prey.

▲ *The forked tongue gives snakes a more acute and directional sense of smell*

The Teeth

All snakes bite, but few are venomous. The word venom means poison. Some snakes have two fangs. These are long, narrow, hollow teeth that lie flat against the roof of the snake's mouth, but the moment a snake sinks its fangs into a prey, muscular pressure releases the venom from a gland located near the eyes. This venom either mobilises the prey or kills it.

▶ *A snake baring its fangs*

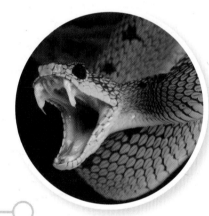

Are all Venomous Snakes Lethal?

Venomous snakes are smart because they do not waste venom on objects they cannot prey on. That is why, although there are about 300 species of venomous snakes, only half are capable of causing lethal harm to human beings. In most cases the human beings are bit in defence as the snake feels that the human being in question is a threat.

Teeth with Another Tale

The non-venomous snakes usually have small sharp teeth which curve backwards. The snake uses these teeth to latch onto a prey, not allowing it to escape as the snake wraps its muscular body around it. Many snakes grow more teeth than required, as some are lost while biting and feeding.

Snake Hug

Most non-venomous snakes and a few venomous ones use constriction as a method to kill their prey. They coil around the prey and suffocate it to death.

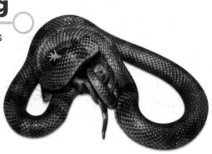

▲ *A snake coiled around a rat*

⊙ Incredible Individuals

Anti-venom is a substance used to treat snake bites against the venom of a particular species of snakes. The first anti-venom was created by Albert Calmette, a scientist working with the Pasteur Institute. It was made against the venom of the Indian cobra, scientifically known as *Naja Naja*.

A King Among Snakes

King cobras are not just one of the most venomous snakes in the world; they can literally 'stand' and rise to the height of a human being. These snakes are found in India, southern China, and Southeast Asia.

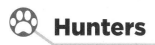 Appearance

King cobras, slender in body, are an average of 12 feet in length, but can reach almost 18 feet. The prominent feature of this species is the presence of 11 large scales on the top of its head. It comes in varied colours and can be black, brown, yellow, or olive green.

The snake's back has crossbar-like sections in white or yellow, while the underside can be monochromatic, with or without the embellishment of bars. The area near the throat is usually light yellow or a brownish cream colour.

◀ *The common stance of a king cobra*

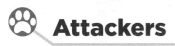 Hunters

King cobras live in forests, fields, and even villages. They can move around at night and in the day time. They are not just seen on land, but also on trees, and in water. They feed on small mammals, bird's eggs, lizards, and even venomous and non-venomous snakes.

Attackers

King cobras do not attack unless they feel threatened. They start out with a loud hiss and spread out their hoods. If the threat persists, they bite. They may not be the most venomous snakes in the world, but the amount of venom they inject into a single bite is enough to kill not just an elephant but almost twenty adult human beings.

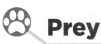 Prey

Human beings have killed so many king cobras for medicine, leather, as well as for entertainment, or in the name of religion, that the poor animal is now on the IUCN list of threatened species.

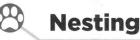 Nesting

On mating, the female of the species lays eggs in a nest. These are the only snakes in the world which don't just build nests but guard them as well. The nest is built by the female using soil, dead leaves, and other buildable materials that she finds on the ground. She coils herself into an arm-like stance to build the nest.

In the Waters

69 species of snakes abound the warm coastal waters of the Pacific and Indian Oceans. However, the span of the yellow-bellied sea snake is much wider, reaching waters of the west coasts of both South and North America.

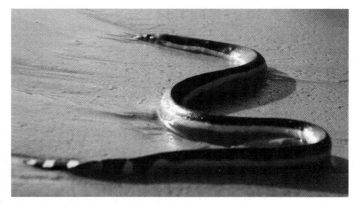

▲ *Yellow-bellied sea snakes have the greatest territory expanse amongst all sea snakes*

Traits

Yellow-bellied sea snakes have flat bodies with oar-like tails and small scales on the back. In a few species, the belly scales are almost absent, making crawling on land impossible for them. They lead most of their lives in water and have elongated lungs almost as long as their bodies.

The sea snakes are known for breathing through the skin. This helps them stay under water for long hours. However, as they have to reach the sea floor for food, they tend to stay in shallow waters, not deeper than 100 feet. They feed on a variety of fish as well as eels.

The Giant of Galapagos

The Galapagos islands can be found in the Pacific Ocean, around 1,000 kilometres off the coast of South America. This network of 19 volcanic islands is home to many rare species of animals. One such species is the giant tortoise or Galapagos tortoise. They are among the longest living vertebrate animals in the world, with an average lifespan of 100 years!

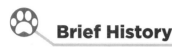

Brief History

The Galapagos Islands were discovered in 1535 by a man named Tomas de Berlanga, who was the bishop of Panama, while travelling to Peru. He saw many tortoises there and named the islands after them, since the Spanish word for these animals is galapagos.

It became famous after many other explorers and even pirates visited the islands. Eventually, it caught the attention of Charles Darwin, who visited the islands in 1835. He encountered almost 15 types of giant tortoises and made a series of observations, which have helped conservationists understand these animals better.

The Shell

The shell of a tortoise is a part of its skeleton. The curved upper part is called the carapace and is supported by the backbone. The lower part, the **plastron**, protects the belly of the animal. The shells are made up of hard bony material, which is covered by a layer of keratin. The shells of the Galapagos tortoises are divided into two types.

The Dome Shell

The dome-shelled tortoises have carapaces angled in such a way that it restricts the extent to which the animal can raise its head. These types tend to live on humid Galapagos islands with abundant vegetation, making it easier to eat food.

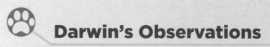

Darwin's Observations

The giant tortoise weighs almost 215 kilograms and is close to 4 feet in length. The tortoise meat was eaten by the inhabitants of the islands and even Charles Darwin tasted it. Island inhabitants would spend around two days hunting a tortoise, but would get enough meat to last them a week! Darwin took home three tortoises for observation.

▼ *Born back in 1832, Jonathan, the oldest living giant tortoise could be 189 years old*

Saddle-shaped Shell

The animals with saddle-shaped shells live on the hotter and drier islands of Galapagos. To survive, their carapaces are angled in such a way, that they can stretch their heads to reach out to vegetation hanging high up.

To Stand and Stare

Galapagos tortoises lead laid-back lives. They bask in the Sun and nap for almost 16 hours a day. The tortoises that live in humid areas eat grass, leaves, and berries. On the other hand, the ones that live in drier regions tend to feed on succulent cactus leaves. They enjoy bathing in water, but can go without food or water for almost a year as they have a slow **metabolism** and massive internal water stores.

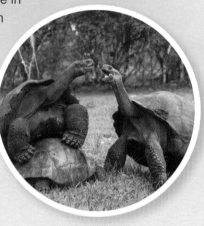

✪ Incredible Individuals

Charles Darwin developed his theory of evolution on the Galapagos islands. He had come to the islands after joining the *HMS Beagle*. The commander of the ship had decided to take along people who would explore the islands and the 22-year-old Darwin had accepted the opportunity.

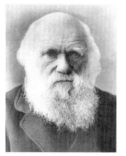
▲ *Charles Darwin*

Before the journey, Darwin was a student at Cambridge, first studying medicine and then divinity. However, his disinterest in his studies embarrassed his father. It was only when Darwin informally studied geology that something sparked within him.

◀ *Male tortoises might stretch out their necks and bite each other to show dominance*

Breeding

During the breeding season, between January to June, males make roaring noises. Females never use their voice. The female lays between 2 to 20 eggs that resemble a tennis ball in size. She digs a hole for the eggs with her hind feet. Once the eggs are covered, she leaves. The eggs hatch after four to eight months, from November to April. The hatchlings are on their own right from the beginning.

Survival

Since Darwin left the islands, the number of the giant tortoises has come down to 10. An estimated 100,000 tortoises have been killed for food in the last 300 years. The main natural predator of the eggs and the hatchlings is the Galapagos hawk. But in case of adult tortoises, illegal hunting and destruction of habitats have made these animals vulnerable to extinction. Conservation efforts by the Charles Darwin Research Centre, under which the eggs and hatchlings are kept in captivity to be released at the right time, are turning out to be helpful.

Sensitive Amphibians

Amphibians partially breathe through their skin. This makes them sensitive to radiation, acid rain, ozone depletion, habitat destruction, pollution, and climatic changes. This is why amphibians are also considered to be indicators of environmental changes.

Playing a Host of Roles

There have been many notions surrounding frogs. Medieval Europeans believed them to be devils. Ancient Egyptians believed that frogs were a symbol of fertility and life. Many children have learned to dissect frogs in their biology classrooms. To scientists, they are a species that have survived millions of years. They are an essential part of the fragile ecosystems of Earth, a prey at times and predator at others. Life without them is impossible!

In the Face of Mass Extinction

Various species of frogs, toads, newts, salamanders, and other amphibians are under threat of extinction because of climatic changes. An example of this is the Chinese giant salamander which has been listed as critically endangered according to the IUCN list. This is because it fills many dinner plates. Yes, because of exploitation for food, there are just a handful of these animals surviving in the wild. The Malagasy rainbow frog that lives in Madagascar too is threatened by the global pet trade.

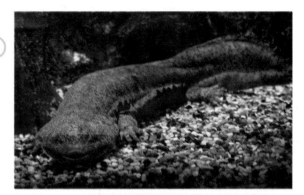

▲ There are five recognised species of the giant salamander

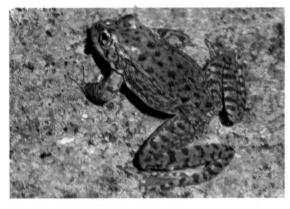

▲ Sierra Nevada mountain yellow-legged frog on a granite rock in the water

Fungal Destruction

High in California's Sierra Nevada, the mountain yellow-legged frogs are dying in big numbers. The reason is amphibian chytrid fungus. It first appeared in 2004 and has killed thousands of animals since then.

The fungus attacks the protein in the amphibian's skin and mouth. This could negatively impact the exchange of gases and the balance of electrolytes, both of which are vital for survival.

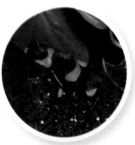

▶ This is the Lehmann's poison frog. It is found in the Colombian jungles of South America. Logging and land development for agriculture has made it critically endangered

▼ The Panamanian golden frog is extinct in the wild. A huge population of this frog has been killed because of the chytrid fungus

Species under Threat

There are many species under threat today, but the Kihansi spray toad and the Panamanian golden frog are some disturbing examples.

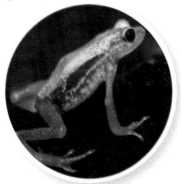

▶ The Kihansi spray toad, as the name suggests, lives amidst the spray of Kihansi and Mhalala waterfalls in the Udzungwa mountains in Tanzania. It is critically endangered

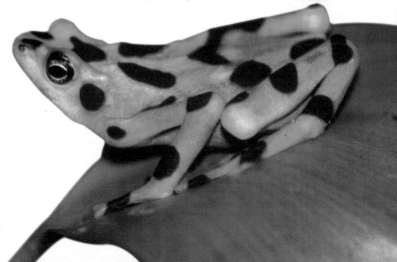

▶ *Black mambas are adapted to live both on the ground and on trees, which they climb easily*

The Venomous Black Mamba

Snakes that can inject venom into their prey are called venomous snakes. Some snakes can also harm human beings with their venom. The substance is poisonous and dangerous. Anti-venom is the cure for venom. Scientists have come up with several anti-venoms by studying snakes and experimenting with their venom.

🐾 Black Mamba

The black mamba is considered to be one of the deadliest snakes of Africa. It is found in the grassy areas and hills of the continent's southern and eastern parts. It is a quick, aggressive, and extremely venomous snake.

The black mamba is not black in colour. It is actually brown! But it gets its name from the blue-black colour found inside its mouth, which it opens wide when threatened. It is Africa's longest venomous snake, reaching almost up to 9 feet in length on an average. It is also one of the fastest snakes in the world and can move at a speed of 20 kmph.

For its aggressive nature, the black mamba is shy. It prefers escape to confrontation. However, if it does feel threatened, it may raise its body to almost one-third of its length and open its mouth to let out a loud hiss. The snake shows its true colours if the threat persists. It attacks multiple times with its fangs, injecting its lethal venom each time.

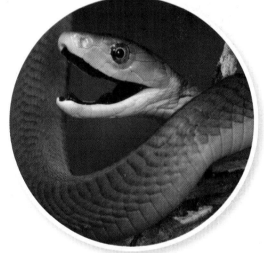

▲ *The brown colour of the black mamba helps the snake camouflage in its surroundings*

🐾 Potent Venom

Black mamba's venom is a **neurotoxin** that paralyses the prey, killing it eventually. If the human beings who are bit do not get the anti-venom immediately, they might die within 20 minutes of the attack. Every year it is responsible for numerous deaths in its home ground, however, some legends and rumours falsely exaggerate these numbers even more.

It is possible that the legends were influenced by the fact that in many rural areas where the black mamba strikes, the **antidote** is not still easily available. Interestingly, recent research shows that black-mamba venom could be more effective than morphine as a painkiller.

This snake is usually found near termite hills. It is either here or in tree hollows that it lays its eggs. It feeds on small mammals and birds.

💡 Isn't It Amazing!

India is often associated with snake charmers. While it is wrong and offensive to stereotype a country in such a way, snake charmers do exist and offer their services as entertainment. They play music and pretend that the snake is dancing to their tune, though in reality, snakes cannot hear very well. The snake charmers are often semi-nomadic and carry king cobras with them. They never harm the animal since it is their source of livelihood. So, if a snake enters a home in a village, they might be the first to be called to remove it.

Activate Defence Mode

Reptiles and amphibians aggressively prey on animals and defend themselves with ease. Many small reptiles fall prey to carnivorous birds, mammals, and even larger reptiles. To protect themselves from danger, small reptiles such as lizards, snakes, and turtles have devised interesting methods of defence. Similarly, amphibians also have special adaptations that keep them safe.

🐾 Ball Up!

The armadillo girdled lizard is found in South Africa. This animal has a unique method of defence. The moment it senses danger, it curls its body into the shape of a ball by holding its tail in its mouth. For attackers, such as snakes, it becomes difficult to swallow the armadillo girdled lizard, not just because they do not know how to take the ball into their mouth, but also because it has a hard, bony covering, and a spiny tail and head. The lizard remains in this shape till the danger passes.

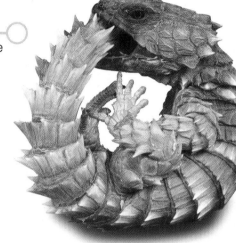

▶ *An armadillo girdled lizard in the defence pose*

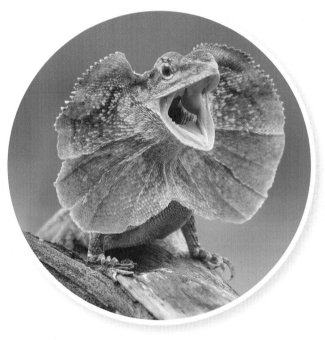

▲ *The Australian frilled lizards are threatened by birds, dingoes, and snakes*

🐾 A Frilled Fight

The Australian frilled lizard uses many tactics to scare off its predators, such as opening its mouth wide, which causes the skin flap to open on both sides of its mouth, making it appear like the lizard has a frilled collar. It also lashes its tail back and forth and makes hissing sounds.

🐾 The Mimic

Scarlet kingsnakes are a smart variety. As part of a defence mechanism called 'mimicry', these harmless snakes sport bright colours similar to the venomous coral snake. Seeing the colours, predators mistake them for the dangerous coral snakes and stay away.

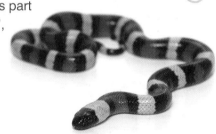

▲ *These snakes are around 30 to 50 centimetres in length*

🐾 Hognose

Hognose snakes feign death if threatened. They roll on their backsides and hang their mouths open. They also emit smells similar to decaying flesh. The predator believes that the snake has been poisoned or diseased and moves away.

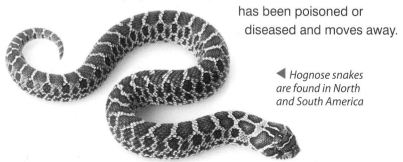

◀ *Hognose snakes are found in North and South America*

👤 In Real Life

Hognose snakes have mild venom, but they are not constrictors. They swallow their prey (like toads) whole. Their venom is not toxic to human beings. They tend to be relatively calm and do not bite trainers. Hognose snakes are shy, so their first defence is to hide from their predators. They hide in burrows or leaves. They are often taken captive and are easy to care for.

🐾 Hinge-back Tortoise

Apart from stiff, bony shells which are the first line of defence in tortoises, few species also have hinges on the shell. When threatened, the hinges allow the front and back of the animal to close tightly, protecting its soft body parts. Not just this, the hinges also give a painful pinch to the predator.

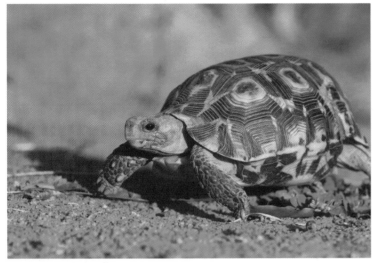

▲ *The hinge-back tortoise likes to look for water underground by burying its head into the land when the water is sparse*

⊕ Incredible Individuals

In Malaysia, there was a famous snake charmer named Ali Khan Samsuddin. He was nicknamed 'King of the Snakes'. Often during his exhilarating shows, he was seen kissing snakes like the king cobra. He once lived in a glass cage with 400 snakes for 40 days. When he was 21, he was first bit by a king cobra but survived. Then again at the age of 48, he was bit by another king cobra, leading to his demise.

🐾 A Horned Defence

Thorny devils are adapted to the Australian outback heat. They have moisture-attracting grooves between the scales. During nights, when dew condenses on their bodies, the grooves take in the moisture and send it to the mouth. This helps them survive harsh climates.

These lizards have prickly horns protruding from their skin. They protect the lizard from being eaten, as the predator stays away seeing the horns. If this does not work, they squirt out blood from tiny vessels near their eyes to scare off the attacker.

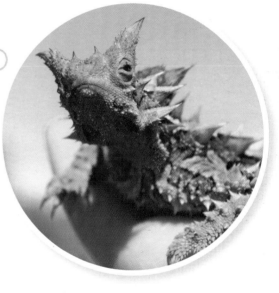

▲ *Thorny devils survive on ants*

🐾 Common Snapping Turtle

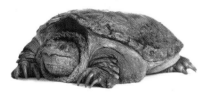

Common snapping turtles often remain buried in muddied shallow waters. They are not aggressive in water, but on land they move forcefully towards the attacker and try snapping their mouths aggressively.

▲ *Do not be fooled by its appearance, a turtle can have a sharp bite*

▼ *These lizards have grey, brown or black skin*

🐾 Five-lined Skink

The five-lined skink wriggles its tail to distract predators. The vertebrae of their tails have special fracture points. If pulled from these points, the tail falls off. The attacker's attention goes to the still-wriggling tail. It lets the lizard out of its mouth and makes a grab for the tail. The lizard escapes and eventually grows a new tail.

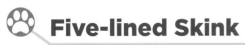

Home Is Where the Habitat Is

Almost all organisms on this planet have homes. There are places that reptiles and amphibians inhabit because they suit their lifestyles the best. These habitats provide them with food, water, and shelter as per their needs. Reptiles and amphibians populate the many places marked on the map below, where they share their homes with other animals.

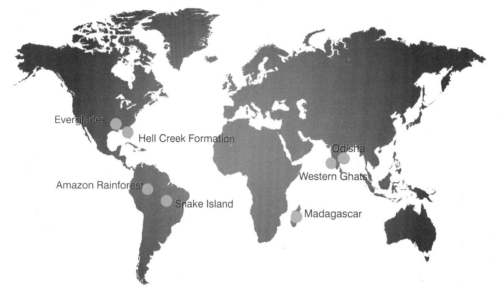

🐾 Amazon Rainforest (South America)

The Amazon River is home to one of the last surviving rainforests in the world. It has abundant trees, swamps, rivulets, and streams for amphibians to live comfortably.

There are many varieties of frogs in the Amazon River. The giant cane toad is a large species that has made its home here. Its skin secretes a toxin so potent that if a cat or dog holds it in its mouth, the animal will die.

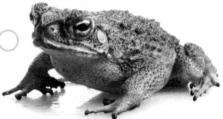

▲ *The largest cane toad was 53.9 centimetres long when stretched from snout to tail, and weighed 2.65 kilograms*

🐾 Western Ghats (India)

Western Ghats lie over the long western coastline of India. They are an ecological treat and are considered one of the eight 'hotspots' of biological diversity around the world. The area is home to at least 325 varieties of threatened plants, mammals, fish, amphibians, and birds.

New species are often discovered here. In 2016, two new species of leaping frogs were discovered here. One is *Indirana paramakri*; it was found on wet rocks and leaves near streams in Kerala. The species is reddish brown with a distinctive snout and unique toe webbing. The other one, *Indirana bhadrai*, is light brown.

▲ *Western Ghats*

🐾 Everglades (USA)

Also called the 'Big Swamp', the Everglades are wetlands of Florida. They are a World Heritage Site. The Everglades are also called the 'river of grass', because of unending miles of sawgrass, at times so thick that one forgets there is water beneath, or *'pahayokee'* (grassy water), as it is called by the Native Americans.

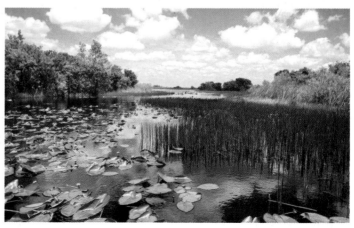

▲ *The grassy waters of the Everglades*

🐾 Snake Island (Brazil)

Off the coast of the city of Sao Paulo lies an island which could be considered the deadliest island in the world. Scientists estimate that around 4,000 snakes inhabit this tiny island. No wonder it is called so.

Here resides the golden lancehead viper, considered to be one of the most venomous pit vipers in the world. Its venom is supposed to be more potent than that of any mainland species.

How was this deadly island created? Once upon a time, it was attached to mainland Brazil, but rising sea levels separated it from the mainland. The snakes there were able to multiply because of the lack of any ground predators.

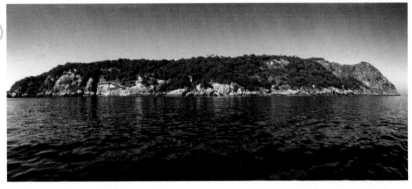

▲ *Snake Island is called Ilha de Queimada Grande*

▶ *Behold the deadly and toxic golden lancehead viper*

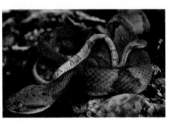

🐾 Hell Creek Formation (USA)

The first-ever *Tyrannosaurus rex* fossil was discovered in 1902 by a palaeontologist named Barnum Brown at Hell Creek Formation in Montana. The fossil belonged to the Cretaceous Age, about 75 million years ago. Since then, several fossils of various dinosaurs have been discovered in this area. To name a few, we have the *Triceratops*, *Edmontosaurus* and *Ankylosaurus*. The entire region was a wet swampy land where dinosaurs roamed freely. To really experience the region's bounty, one can take part in excavation programmes at Hell Creek! All we need is a guide, a digging supervisor and a calm mind to make sure no fossil is damaged in the process.

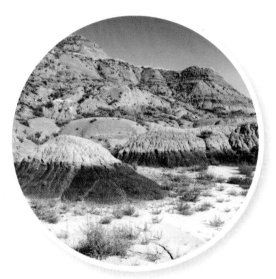

▲ *Hell Creek is sometimes referred to as 'badlands' because it is barren, eroded, and almost devoid of vegetation*

🐾 Odisha (India)

Olive ridley turtles are found in warm waters of the three oceans, the Atlantic, Pacific, and Indian. They are named so because of the greenish colour of their skin and carapace. These reptiles are small, measuring about 2 feet in length.

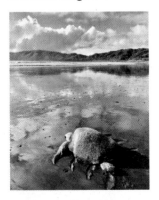

The female turtles migrate thousands of kilometres to lay eggs. One such site is the coastline of Odisha in India. Females visit it in large numbers, making it a mass nesting site.

▲ *To ensure that some will hatch, live, and make it to adulthood, they lay 120–150 eggs at a time!*

🐾 Madagascar (Africa)

The island of Madagascar is not just home to the world's smallest chameleon, but also to the world's longest, the Parson's chameleon. This reptile can grow almost up to 70 centimetres in length. If you want to see this lizard, you will have to make a trip to the rainforests on the island. These chameleons live on trees there.

They have independently moving eyes and a triangular head similar to other types of chameleons. A long tail is used for gripping branches. The chameleon's long, sticky tongue helps it capture insects.

Like most chameleons, Parson's too changes colour not just as camouflage, but also based on environmental factors such as light and temperature, as well as based on the presence of other chameleons.

▶ *Parson's chameleons are said to be gentle lizards*

Word Check

Birds

Aerodynamic: It means to have qualities which make it possible to move through air easily.

Carrion: It is the decaying flesh of dead animals.

Endangered species: It refers to species where the population is so low, they could soon go extinct.

Hereditary: It refers to something that is passed from generation to generation.

Fossil: It is a bone of an animal, part of a plant, or shell whose shape has been preserved in a rock for a long period of time.

Keratin: It is a fibrous protein that is present on the outer layer of feathers, nails, and hooves.

Mating season: It is a period during which males and females of a species mate most often to produce offspring.

Moulting: It is the process by which birds shed their feathers and replace them with new feathers.

Ornithologist: It refers to a person who is involved in the study of birds.

Ornithology: It refers to the study of birds.

Piscivorous: It refers to birds that eat fish as the staple of their diets.

Ratites: It refers to a group of flightless birds like the ostrich and emu.

Regurgitate: It means to bring up the swallowed food again to the mouth. Some birds do this to feed their young ones.

Species: It refers to a group of closely related living organisms which are like each other and can interbreed to produce offspring.

Insects

Arthropods: They form the largest order of the animal kingdom, mainly consisting of animals with 'jointed' legs.

Bioluminescence: It is the process by which light is emitted from a living organism like a glow-worm or firefly.

Cross pollinators: It refers to sources of pollination of a flower or plant with pollen from another flower or plant.

Defoliation: It is the destruction of leaves.

Ectoparasites: These are parasites that live outside the body of the host.

Elytra: They are the hardened wings of an insect like a beetle or weevil.

Genetically modified: It refers to the process of altering the genetic constituency. Both organisms as well as fruits and vegetables can be genetically modified.

Hibernate: It means to spend days in a state of inactivity, especially during winters when sources of food are minimum, and the weather is not conducive for survival.

Incomplete metamorphosis: Similar to metamorphosis, but here the pupa stage is absent

Metamorphosis: It is the process by which an organism transforms from its younger stage to an adult. After this transformation, the adult does not resemble the young ones from the same species.

Monophagous: It refers to feeding on a single kind of plant or animal.

Moulting: It is the process by which an animal sheds its exoskeleton to regrow a new one.

Nymph: It is the form of an insect that does not transform in appearance as it grows.

Parasitic: It is the practice or behaviour of an organism that depends on exploiting another organism for survival.

Regurgitated: It refers to food that is swallowed by animals and then brought up again.

Sericulture: It is the process of rearing silkworms and thereafter producing silk.

Spiracles: The small openings or holes on the exoskeleton that allow an animal to breathe.

Sterile: It refers to an organism that is unable to reproduce.

Stridulating: It means to produce a sharp and shrill sound by rubbing the wings, legs or other body parts together.

Stylets: Thin and needle-like insect mouthparts.

Thyroid: It is a small gland which regulates the growth and development of the body.

Xylophage: It refers to an insect or organism that feeds on wood.

Invertebrates

Cephalisation: It refers to the presence of sense organs and brain in the upper part of the body.

Chitinous: It refers to animals with a semi-transparent substance which forms part of the exoskeleton in arthropods.

Coelom: It is the fluid-filled body cavity which acts as a cushion for the internal organs.

Enzymes: They are substances produced by living organisms which bring about a biochemical reaction.

Hermaphrodites: It means an organism has both male and female sex organs.

Hydrostatic: It is associated with fluids and their pressure.

Myriapods: It is an arthropod group; the animals have elongated bodies with numerous legs.

Pentamerous: It means that the parts of the body are arranged in a group of five.

Photosynthesis: It is the process by which green plants prepare food in the presence of sunlight and a pigment called chlorophyll that is present in the leaves of plants. The plants also need carbon dioxide and water to release energy and oxygen.

Polyp: It is an individual coral organism.

Single-celled bacteria: This bacteria has only one functional and structural unit.

Thorax: It is the middle section in an insect, between the head and abdomen.

Visceral: It refers to the internal organs, especially in the abdominal region.

Mammals

Blowhole: The nostril at the top of a whale or dolphin's head

Blubber: It is the fat in a sea mammal's body that keeps it warm.

Browsing: It refers to animals feeding on vegetation that grows on trees like leaves and twigs from trees.

Carapace: It is the hard, upper shell structure of a mammal like a glyptodont or tortoise.

Diurnal: It refers to animals that are active during the day and rest during the night.

Dorsal: It refers to the upper area or back of an animal.

Echolocation: It is the method of using sound waves and echoes to understand where different objects are placed in a path.

Endothermy: The ability to generate heat and regulate the body temperature internally

Ethologist: It refers to a person involved in ethology—the study of animal behaviour focusing on the patterns that they exhibit in their natural environment.

Foetus: It refers to an unborn vertebrate that is still developing.

Hair follicles: It is a part of the skin formed by padding old cells together. Hair grows from hair follicles.

Incubate: It refers to the process by which birds sit on the eggs that they lay to keep them warm before they hatch.

Marsupials: An animal species whose female lacks enough placenta and has a pouch on the abdomen in which she carries the young to feed and nurture it

Monotreme: It is a mammalian order of egg-laying animals like the duck-billed platypus.

Moult: It means to shed old feathers, skin, or fur.

Nocturnal: It refers to animals that are active during the night and rest during the day.

Omnivorous: It refers to an animal that eats both plants and other animals.

Opposable thumb: It means that the thumb can be held opposite to the other fingers on the hand. Hands with opposable thumbs can form fists to hold objects.

Paleontologist: It refers to a person who studies palaeontology—the branch of science that deals with fossils of dead animals and plants.

Pectoral fins: They are the fins present on either sides of mammals such as dolphins. They reside just behind the mammal's head.

Placenta: It refers to an organ that is temporary. Its function is to join the mother to the foetus in a way that the transfer of oxygen, nutrients, and waste becomes easier.

Savannahs: They are open plains in the tropics that are covered with grass and little trees.

Umbilical cord: It exists in animals that have placenta while giving birth. It is a pipe between the placenta and the developing foetus.

Vertebrates: It refers to animals that have backbones or spinal cords covered with bones.

Viviparous: It refers to a group of animals that reproduce by live birth instead of reproducing by laying eggs.

Marine Animals

Alevin: It is the newly born salmon or trout fish.

Amnion: It is the membrane which encircles the embryo of a mammal, reptile, or bird.

Anadromous: It is a fish that migrates upstream in rivers in order to mate.

Antidote: It is a medicine that fights the effects of a poison.

Ballast: It is an organ that helps an animal (like the fish) maintain its depth in water without sinking or floating.

Calcareous: It is a shell made up of calcium carbonate.

Cartilaginous: It refers to animals that have a skeleton of cartilage, which is a soft connective tissue found in the body.

Catadromous: It means migrating down rivers to the sea to spawn.

Chordate: It refers to an animal that possesses vertebrae and belongs to the large phylum Chordata.

Dormant: It refers to species that are inactive.

Ectotherms: It refers to cold-blooded animals which depend on external heat sources to regulate their body temperature.

Electroreceptive organs: They are special organs in the skin of certain fish, which help them detect electric signals.

Endoskeleton: It is the internal skeleton.

Exoskeleton: It is the hard, external covering that is seen in invertebrate animals.

Gondwana: It is the continent that was formed in the southern hemisphere after the break-up of Pangaea. It later separated to form South America, Africa, Antarctica, Australia, Arabia, and the peninsula of India.

Hermaphrodite: It is a living organism that has both male and female reproduction organs.

Nervous system: It is a network of nerve cells and fibres that carry instructions to and from the different body parts to the brain.

Notochord: It refers to the cartilaginous skeletal rod that supports the body of an animal when it is at the embryonic (developing) stage.

Reptiles & Amphibians

Amphibians: It is a class of animals that are cold-blooded and includes vertebrates such as frogs, toads, newts, salamanders and caecilians. All amphibians are aquatic at the larval stage and have gills. They metamorphise into adults who can move on land and breathe using lungs.

Antidote: It is the medicine given to nullify the effects of poison.

Arthropods: It is a class of invertebrate animals that have an exoskeleton, a segmented body, and paired appendages that are jointed. They are a very diverse group, with around 10 million species worldwide, such as lobsters, spiders, centipedes, many types of insects.

Exoskeleton: It is the hard, external covering seen in invertebrate animals.

Larva: It is a stage in the life of an amphibian or insect where it is completely different from its adult form.

Lobe-finned fish: These fish have a central appendage made up of bones and cartilage in their fins. This is what helped tetrapods walk on land.

Mesozoic Era: It was a period around 65 million years ago when giant dinosaurs, birds and reptiles dominated Earth.

Metabolism: It refers to the chemical reactions that take place within the body of an animal, including digestion and respiration.

Moulting: It is the process by which an animal sheds its exoskeleton and grows another.

Neurotoxin: It is a type of venom that paralyses or stuns the prey.

Plastron: It is the underside of a tortoise or turtle's shell.

Sauropsids: It is a group of amniotic animals that consists of birds and reptiles.

Synapsids: It is the class of animals containing all mammal species.

Tetrapod: It is an animal that possesses four feet.

Triassic takeover: It lasted between 251 and 199 million years ago after the Permian Mass Extinction wiped out most synapsids and sauropsids began to evolve.

a: above, b: below/ bottom, c: centre, f: far, l: left, r: right, t: top, bg: background

Cover

Shutterstock:

Front: FloridaStock; Smit; ilikestudio; Yellow Cat; vladsilver; Nathapol Kongseang; Olena Herz; ArtLovePhoto; cbpix; Kurit afshen; Glass and Nature; Anan Kaewkhammul; Eric Isselee; panor156; maratr; Rich Carey; Grigorev Mikhail; Alex Staroseltsev; Jiang Zhongyan; Inachis Projekt; Thetor.P

Back: Mike Truchon; Eric Isselee; Gladkova Svetlana; irin-k; Protasov AN; Eric Isselee; Sarunyu_foto; Eric Isselee; Hintau Aliaksei; TobyG

Birds

Shutterstock: Mike Truchon; Roger Clark ARPS; Drakuliren; Glass and Nature; clarst5; TobyG; FloridaStock; jo Crebbin; Axel Alvarez; Tracy Starr; Francois Loubser; Eric Isselee; Narupon Nimpaiboon; Krakenimages.com

Inside

Shutterstock: 3b/Jesse Nguyen; 3tbg/Andy Vinnikov; 4tr/Warpaint; 4cl/Herschel Hoffmeyer; 5tc/AKKHARAT JARUSILAWONG; 5b/Michael Rosskothen; 5cr/Michael Rosskothen; 6b/Mriya Wildlife; 6c/MustafaNC; 6&7c/Eric Isselee; 6&7bg/luck luckyfarm; 6/peacefoo; 7tr/ehtesham; 7b/Narupon Nimpaiboon; 8cl/FloridaStock; 8bl/Daniel_Kay; 9tr/Mike Truchon; 9tl/Eric Isselee; 9cr/Tracy Starr; 9br1/Four Oaks; 9br2/Rocky Grimes; 9bl/Eric Isselee; 10tr/Patthana Nirangkul; 10cl/Jesus Giraldo Gutierrez; 10br/Vladimir Soltys; 11tr/Juho Salo; 11cl/Sue Harper Photography; 11br/Koraysa; 11br/Jan Zoetekouw; 12t/WitR; 12cl/Sergey Uryadnikov; 12bc/Valentina Photo; 12br/maratr; 13tr/Yuliya Derbisheva VLG; 13tr1/Rudmer Zwerver; 13c/Melinda Nagy; 13br/hanif66; 14tc/clarst5; 14tr/Mike Truchon; 14cr/Annette Shaff; 14bl/ANCH; 14bl1/Bonnie Taylor Barry; 14br1/Fexel; 15tr/Rob Christiaans; 15cr/Hayley Crews; 15bl/Tim Zurowski; 15br/Stubblefield Photography; 16tl/Tracy Starr; 16cl/Ger Bosma Photos; 16br/Narupon Nimpaiboon; 16br1/vyasphoto; 17tr/Mike Truchon; 17crl/Ondrej Prosicky; 17br/Denise LaPerriere; 18tr/serkan mutan; 18&19c/nadtytok; 18cl/irin-k; 18br/Rudmer Zwerver; 19tr/Rosa Jay; 19cr/Jesse Nguyen; 20tl/TobyG; 20bl/Chad Wright Photography; 20&21/Le Do; 21tl/tristan tan; 21cr1/Kerry Hargrove; 21cr2/Kerry Hargrove; 21br/photomaster; 22tc/Patthana Nirangkul; 22cl/Javier Valladares; 22cr/Maciej Olszewski; 22bl/Francois Loubser; 23bl/colacat; 23bc/Ondrej Prosicky; 23bc2/Christian Musat; 23bc3/Anastasiia Petrych; 23br/Aaron Amat; 23br1/picturepartners; 24tc/Martin Mecnarowski; 24tr/finchfocus; 24cl1/Cathy Withers-Clarke; 24cl/meunierd; 24cr/Drakuliren; 24cr1/Simun Ascic; 24&25bg/Chayatorn Laorattanavech; 24&25bg/sumroeng chinnapan; 25tc/jo Crebbin; 25tc1/Nick Pecker; 25tr/Vishnevskiy Vasily; 25cl/Sergey Uryadnikov; 25bc/Joseph Sohm; 26cr/Stacey Arsenault; 26cl/Ana Gram; 26bl/Devin Koob; 26br/Roger Clark ARPS; 27cr/aarondfrench; 27cl/zffoto; 27br/Dr Ajay Kumar Singh; 27tr/Coatesy; 27tc/Wang LiQiang; 28tr/javarman; 28c/Roger Clark ARPS; 28bl/Ondrej Prosicky; 28&29bg/2j architecture; 29tl/Iurii Kazakov; 29tr/Sergey Uryadnikov; 29cr/vladsilver; 29br/nwdph; 30br/Michael Shake; 30b/Viktor Loki; 31tr/Wang LiQiang; 31c/Anna Moskvina; 31br/violetkaipa;

Insects

Shutterstock: alslutsky; Protasov AN; Eric Isselee; irin-k; Mr. SUTTIPON YAKHAM; Hintau Aliaksei; chakkrachai nicharat; arka38; ArtLovePhoto; Alex Staroseltsev; suns07butterfly; Elliotte Rusty Harold; Evgeniy Ayupov; Luc Pouliot; anat chant; Anton Kozyrev; schankz; Lukas Gojda

Inside

Shutterstock: 33tr/Andy Vinnikov; 3b/Awei; 4&5tc/anat chant; 4bl/tienduc1103; 5cr/Radu Bercan; 5c/Luc Pouliot; 6tr/Brett Hondow; 6cr/Mr. SUTTIPON YAKHAM; 6bl/Tomasz Klejdysz; 6br/NaMaKuKi; 7tr/Anton Kozyrev; 7cl/Aleksey Stemmer; 7br/Vitalii Hulai; 8tr/Alex Staroseltsev; 8cl/Vaclav Volrab; 8cr/Muhammad Naaim; 8b/Lukas Gojda; 9tr/khlungcenter; 9bl/WUT.ANUNAI; 10tr/BOONCHUAY PROMJIAM; 10bl/majeczka; 10br/Protasov AN; 11tr/Oleg1824; 11tl/Cosmin Manci; 11cr/Mark Brandon; 11bl/ArchMan; 11br/Leena Robinson; 12c/Nicolas Primola; 12cr/1st-ArtZone; 12cr1/KanphotoSS; 12bl/Chekaramit; 13tr/Leena Robinson; 13bl/ilikestudio; 14&15c/Eric Isselee; 14br/PetrP; 14bl/JD Phote; 15cr/D L Kugler; 16cl/DWI YULIANTO; 16bl/Sebastian Janicki; 17tl/Hawk777; 17cr/Hintau Aliaksei; 17bc/Helen Cradduck; 18tr/Ondrej Prosicky; 18bl/Evgeniy Ayupov; 19tr/Stephane Bidouze; 19bl/Eric Isselee; 19br/Mark Brandon; 20tr/arka38; 20bl/Vladimir Wrangel; 20br/aaabbbccc; 21tr/Cosmin Manci; 21bl/D. Kucharski K. Kucharska; 21br/Jaco Visser; 22tr/Africa Studio; 22bl/New Africa; 24br/irin-k; 23t&24b/irin-k; 22&23 tc/Daniel Prudek; 23t/enterphoto; 24tr/paula french; 24bl/Tsekhmister; 25tr/Protasov AN; 25cr/moomsabuy; 25bl/Songsak P; 25bc/GreenTree; 26tr/frank60; 26bl/Achkin; 27cl/tozzimr; 27br/Andrey Pavlov; 27b1/Eric Isselee; 27b2/Eric Isselee; 27b3/Eric Isselee; 28cl/Rostasedlacek; 28cr/Marek Poplawski; 28bc/chakkrachai nicharat; 29tr/Pan Xunbin; 29cl/Chaikom; 30tr/frank60; 30bc/ArtLovePhoto; 31tr/Rav Kark; 31cr/Eric Isselee; 31bl/Protasov AN

Wikimedia Commons: 30br/File:Charles Laveran nobel.jpg/Laveran.jpg: Eugène Pirou (1841–1909)derivative work: Materialscientist, Public domain, via Wikimedia Commons/ wikimedia commons

Invertebrates

Shutterstock: Andrew Burgess; Kletr; Studioimagen73; PetlinDmitry; Volosina; Louella938; ppl; Knorre; Jiang Zhongyan; Yutthasart Yanakornsiri; Smit; Olena Herz; arka38; photomaster; Luca Santilli; Lotus Images; Rattiya Thongdumhyu; yothinpi; ileana_bt; Onur ERSIN;

Inside

Shutterstock: 3tr/By Andy Vinnikov; 3b/By John A. Anderson; 4tr/By Benny Marty; 4cl/By Cheng Wei; 4br/By Eugen Thome; 5tr/By Esteban De Armas; 5cl/By AuntSpray; 6tl/By Roblan; 6tl1/By Andrew Burgess; 6bl/By Michal Hykel; 7tr/By Kristine Reed; 7cl/By Andrew Burgess; 8cl/By Louella938; 8cr/By Choksawatdikorn; 8cr1/By Levent Konuk; 8bl/By Olena Herz; 8bl1/By arka38; 8bl2/By arka38; 8br/By Rattiya Thongdumhyu; 9tl/By Studioimagen73; 9tl1/By Aleksandar Dickov; 9tl2/By Volosina; 9tl3/By Jiang Zhongyan; 9bl/By Nataly Studio; 9bl/By jps; 9bl/By Yutthasart Yanakornsiri; 9cr1/By Lotus Images; 9cr2/By Lotus Images; 9cr3/By anat chant; 9cr4/By Onur ERSIN; 9bl1/By ileana_bt; 9bl2/By Anton Starikov; 9bl3/By CY BAI; 9bl4/By Knorre; 10tr/By cbpix; 10cl/By Dr Morley Read; 10bl/By PetlinDmitry; 10br/By Daleen Loest; 11tr/By Choksawatdikorn; 11cr/By JIANG HONGYAN; 11br/By Aleksey Stemmer; 12tr/By Teguh Tirtaputra; 12cr/By Krzysztof Bargiel; 12bl/By Henrik Larsson; 12br/By NatureDiver; 13tr/By NatalieJean; 13cr/By yothinpi; 13bl/By Henk Bogaard; 14bl/By Damsea; 14&15b /By DJ Mattaar; 15b/By Choksawatdikorn; 15br/By Richard Whitcombe; 16br/By Ethan Daniels; 17tl/By Ethan Daniels; 17br/By V_E; 18tr/By Juan Gaertner; 18cr/By Blamb; 18bc/By Bannasak Krokdeaw; 19cr2/By Tridsanu Thopet; 19cr1/By Kateryna Kon; 19cl/By Protasov AN; 19bl/By D. Kucharski K. Kucharska; 19br/By Lontano; 20tl/By Kletr; 20cr/By Andrey Armyagov; 20br/By Ivan Marjanovic; 21tr/By LedyX; 21cr/By Guillermo Guerao Serra; 21bl/By Kuttelvaserova Stuchelova; 21br/By reptiles4all; 22&23c/By JIANG HONGYAN; 22cl/By feathercollector; 22br/By Isabelle van Mierlo; 23tr1/By Cassidy Scott; 23tr2/By Cassidy Scott; 24tr/By ppl; 24cr/By Alexandr Grant; 24bl/By Witaya Proadtayakogool; 25tr/By piya saisawatdikul; 25cl/By Vitalii Hulai; 25br/By photowind; 26tr/By Process; 26bl/By itor; 26br/By Mikhail Kovalev; 27cr/By Luca Santilli; 27bl/By JimboMcKimbo; 27br/By KYTan; 28tr/By Jan Danek jdm.foto; 28cl/By photomaster; 28br/By Cathy Keifer; 29tr/By cyrrpit; 29cr/By Amith Nag; 29bl/By Protasov AN; 29br/By Dr Morley Read; 30&31c/By Smit; 30bl/ By Ethan Daniels; 31tr/By koi88; 31bl/By XAOC; 31br/By Sergey Zuenok;

Mammals

Marine Animals

Reptiles & Amphibians